100 ORGANIC SKINCARE RECIPES:

Major Prophet PD John
P.O. BOX 4016
Mwanza - Tanzania
Phone number:
+255 762 415 790/ +255 759 204 744
Yohanayona3@gmail.com
www.hl centre.info

ISBN : 9798329716429
First edition ©2024.
Imprint: Independently published

Chief Editor:
Josia pd John
josiajohn735@gmail.com
Dar es salaam - Tanzania
Tel: +255 758588127/ +255 693522834

"100 Organic Skincare Recipes:

Dedication

To my dearest friend, nature, whose boundless beauty and wisdom have inspired every page of this book. Thank you for providing the nourishing ingredients that have allowed us to create these 100 organic skincare recipes. May we continue to learn from your timeless secrets and cherish the natural beauty you bestow upon us all.

Preface

In the pursuit of beauty, we often find ourselves drawn to the shelves of stores filled with an array of skincare products, each promising transformative results. These products, however, often come at a cost—both to our wallets and to the environment. The realization that the best ingredients for our skin are found in nature itself is what led to the creation of this book, *"100 Organic Skincare Recipes: A Comprehensive Guide to Natural Beauty."*

The journey to this book's creation has been a labor of love, driven by a passion for harnessing the power of nature to enhance our skin's health and radiance. As we embarked on this endeavor, we were guided by a profound appreciation for the Earth's abundant offerings and a deep desire to share the knowledge of crafting organic skincare products with you.

Before we delve into the pages of this comprehensive guide, we want to express our gratitude through the dedication in the front of this book. It is a tribute to the source of our inspiration—the natural world and its wonders.

Within these pages, you will discover not only one hundred meticulously crafted organic skincare recipes but also a deeper understanding of the beauty and wisdom nature holds. We invite you to embrace the principles of natural beauty, sustainability, and self-care as you explore the recipes and guidance we've prepared for you.

Whether you're seeking a gentle cleanser for your face, a luxurious body lotion, or a soothing remedy for skin ailments, we have strived to provide a diverse array of recipes to meet your skincare needs. Each recipe has been thoughtfully formulated using organic, readily available ingredients, and we've included options for customization to suit your unique skin type and preferences.

As you embark on this journey with us, remember that the true essence of beauty lies not only in the radiant glow of your skin but also in the knowledge that you are caring for yourself and the planet simultaneously. By choosing organic skincare, you are making a conscious decision to honor the Earth, promote sustainability, and prioritize your well-being.

We encourage you to experiment, create, and adapt these recipes to suit your individual needs and preferences. By doing so, you'll not only enhance your natural beauty but also cultivate a deeper connection with the natural world.

Thank you for joining us on this exploration of organic skincare, and may the pages that follow serve as a source of inspiration, empowerment, and rejuvenation as you embark on your path to embracing the beauty of nature.

With heartfelt gratitude,

[Prophet PD John]

Acknowledgments

Creating a book of this magnitude is a collaborative effort, and we are deeply grateful to the individuals and sources that have contributed to the realization of *"100 Organic Skincare Recipes: A Comprehensive Guide to Natural Beauty."* This book would not have been possible without their support, expertise, and inspiration.

We extend our heartfelt thanks to:

1. **Mother Nature:** The ultimate source of inspiration for this book. Thank you for providing us with the incredible ingredients and wisdom that make organic skincare possible.

2. **Family and Friends:** To our loved ones who supported us throughout this journey, providing

encouragement, patience, and understanding during countless hours of recipe testing and writing.

3. **Our Readers:** You, the readers, are the reason we embarked on this project. Your enthusiasm for natural beauty and organic skincare fuels our passion for sharing this knowledge.

4. **Our Editors and Proofreaders:** Your meticulous attention to detail and commitment to clarity have been invaluable in ensuring the quality of this book.

5. **Contributing Experts:** We'd like to express our gratitude to the skincare experts and herbalists who generously shared their knowledge and insights, enriching the content of this book.

6. **Sustainability Advocates:** Those dedicated to promoting eco-conscious living and sustainable practices have inspired us to include sections on ethical and sustainable skincare choices.

7. **Artists and Designers:** Thank you for crafting the visually appealing elements of this book that enhance the overall reading experience.

8. **Publishing Team:** To our publishers, designers, and everyone involved in bringing this book to life and making it available to readers worldwide, we extend our heartfelt appreciation.

9. **Mother Earth:** Once more, we acknowledge our planet for her abundance and for the wisdom she imparts. May we all strive to be better stewards of her resources.

This book is a testament to the beauty of collaboration and the belief that, by harnessing the gifts of the natural world, we can enhance our well-being while treading lightly on the Earth. Our gratitude to all who have played a part in this endeavor is immeasurable.

With sincere thanks,

[Prophet PD John]

Table of Contents

Chapter I:

Introduction

A. The Benefits of Organic Skincare

In the pursuit of health and beauty, it is written in the Book of Genesis, ***"And God saw everything that he had made, and behold, it was very good"*** **(Genesis 1:31, ESV).** This ancient wisdom reminds us that the natural world, including the plants and herbs that grace our Earth, carries inherent goodness. Organic skincare harnesses this goodness, offering numerous benefits for our skin. As we explore the recipes within these pages, we draw inspiration from the divine wisdom found in the creation of all things.

B. Why Make Your Own Skincare Products?

"And God said, 'See, I have given you every herb that yields seed which is on the face of all the earth, and every tree whose fruit yields seed; to you it shall be for food.'" **(Genesis 1:29, NKJV).** This verse underscores the abundance of the Earth's offerings. Making your own skincare products allows you to harness the nourishing power of these herbs and plants, free from harmful additives. In doing so, you honor the gift of creation and take charge of what you apply to your skin, aligning with the divine intention.

C. How to Use This Book

As you embark on this journey of discovering and creating organic skincare, consider the wisdom of **Proverbs 2:6 (NIV):** *"For the Lord gives wisdom; from his mouth come knowledge and understanding."* In this book, you will find not only recipes but also knowledge and understanding of organic skincare. Each section is carefully crafted to guide you on your path to natural beauty:

- Chapter 1 explores the benefits of organic skincare, rooted in the wisdom of God's creation.

- Chapter 2 delves into essential tools and ingredients, providing you with the knowledge needed for successful skincare creations.

- Subsequent chapters offer a diverse array of recipes, inspired by the bountiful Earth and designed to enhance your well-being.

As you journey through this comprehensive guide, may you find wisdom, inspiration, and a deeper connection to the natural world, all in alignment with the divine plan.

"For everything created by God is good, and nothing is to be rejected if it is received with thanksgiving" **(1 Timothy 4:4, ESV).** Let this book be your guide to receiving the goodness of organic skincare with gratitude and reverence for the Creator's divine design.

Chapter II:

Understanding Organic Skincare

A. What Makes Skincare Products Organic?

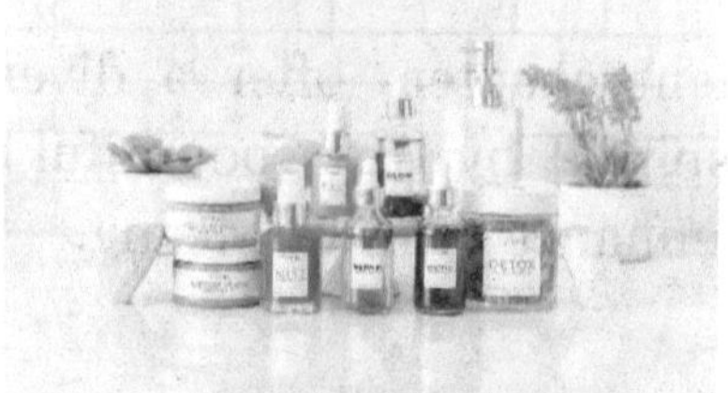

In today's world, where the pursuit of natural and organic lifestyles has gained significant momentum, the term ***"organic"*** has become a buzzword in various industries, including skincare. But what exactly does it mean when we refer to skincare products as ***"organic"?*** In this chapter, we will delve deep into the concept of organic skincare, exploring the intricacies of what makes a skincare product truly organic.

1. Organic Certification: A Foundation of Trust

At the heart of organic skincare lies the concept of certification. Organic skincare products are not merely those that claim to be natural; they undergo a rigorous certification process to earn the "organic" label. This process involves adherence to strict standards set by certifying bodies, which can vary by region. In the United States, for example, the USDA (United States Department of Agriculture) sets standards for organic products. In the European Union, there are different certification bodies.

Organic certification encompasses various aspects, including the sourcing of raw materials, cultivation practices, and manufacturing processes. To be certified as organic, skincare products must meet specific criteria, such as:

- **Use of Organic Ingredients:** The primary ingredients used in the product must be grown and harvested without synthetic pesticides, herbicides, or genetically modified organisms (GMOs). This ensures that the plant-based components of the product are in alignment with organic farming principles.

- **Environmental Sustainability:** Organic skincare production often emphasizes sustainability and eco-friendliness. This includes responsible water use, energy efficiency, and minimizing waste generation.

- **Animal Welfare:** Many organic certifications also have guidelines that promote cruelty-free practices, ensuring that products are not tested on animals.

- **Transparency:** Brands seeking organic certification must provide detailed records of their ingredient sourcing, manufacturing processes, and quality control measures. This transparency fosters trust between consumers and producers.

2. The Importance of Natural Ingredients

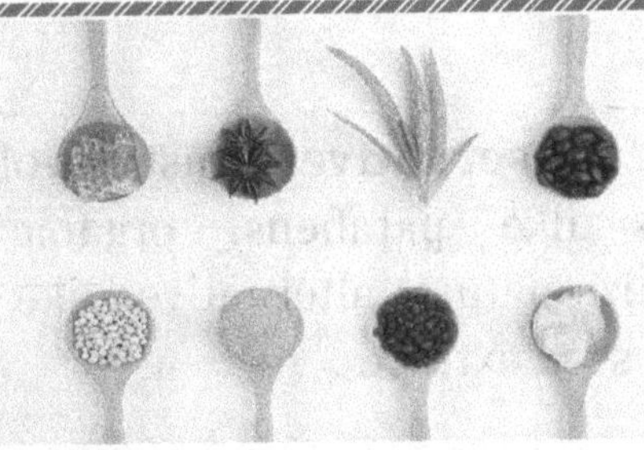

"And God said, 'Let the earth bring forth grass, the herb yielding seed, and the fruit tree yielding fruit after his kind, whose seed is in itself, upon the earth: and it was so.'" **(Genesis 1:11, KJV).** The divine wisdom in this verse underscores the intrinsic value of natural ingredients in skincare. Organic skincare products prioritize the use of botanical and natural ingredients, shunning synthetic and potentially harmful chemicals.

- **Botanical Extracts:** Organic skincare often incorporates plant-based extracts, such as aloe vera, chamomile, and lavender, renowned for their soothing and rejuvenating properties.

- **Essential Oils:** These potent oils, extracted from plants, provide aromatic and therapeutic benefits. Examples include lavender, tea tree, and rosehip oil.

- Natural Preservatives: Instead of synthetic preservatives like parabens, organic skincare products utilize natural alternatives like vitamin E or grapefruit seed extract.

3. Transparency and Labeling

To assist consumers in making informed choices, regulatory bodies often require that organic skincare products display their certification logos and provide ingredient lists. Understanding product labels and ingredient lists empowers consumers to discern genuine organic products from those that may only carry partial organic ingredients.

4. The Impact on Skin and the Environment

Organic skincare products are celebrated not only for what they exclude *(synthetic chemicals)* but also for what they include (natural goodness). When applied to the skin, these products can provide a range of benefits, such as reduced risk of irritation and enhanced hydration. Moreover, by supporting organic farming practices, these products contribute to a healthier planet, promoting soil fertility, biodiversity, and reduced chemical runoff.

In essence, what makes skincare products organic is a combination of certification, natural ingredients, transparency, and ethical practices. By understanding these elements, you'll be better equipped to navigate the world of organic skincare and make choices that align with your values and promote the well-being of both your skin and the environment.

B. The Importance of Natural Ingredients

"And God said, 'Let the earth bring forth grass, the herb yielding seed, and the fruit tree yielding fruit after his kind, whose seed is in itself, upon the earth: and it was so.'" **(Genesis 1:11, KJV).** In these divine words, we find the fundamental

principle that underscores the importance of natural ingredients in skincare. Nature, in its wisdom, has provided an abundance of botanical treasures that have nourished and healed humanity for centuries. Understanding the significance of these natural ingredients in skincare is key to appreciating the holistic benefits they offer.

1. Harmony with Human Biology

Natural ingredients in skincare products resonate with our bodies in a way that synthetic chemicals often cannot. The composition of natural ingredients, whether plant extracts or essential oils, often mirrors the chemical composition of our skin. This harmony can lead to better absorption and compatibility, reducing the risk of skin irritation and allergies.

2. Nutrient-Rich Formulations

Natural ingredients are teeming with nutrients, antioxidants, vitamins, and minerals that promote skin health. For instance, aloe vera, known as the *"plant of immortality,"* contains compounds that soothe and hydrate the skin, while rosehip oil, abundant in ***vitamin C,*** supports collagen production and skin brightening. These natural gifts provide a wealth of benefits, from moisturizing and nourishing to protecting against environmental stressors.

3. Gentle and Nourishing

*"The earth brought forth vegetation, plants yielding seed according to their own kinds, and trees bearing fruit in which is their seed, each according to its kind." **(Genesis 1:12, ESV).*** Just as each plant yields fruits and seeds according to its kind, natural ingredients deliver specific skincare benefits according to their unique properties. For instance:

- Chamomile and calendula offer soothing properties, making them ideal for sensitive or irritated skin.

- Tea tree oil is celebrated for its antibacterial and acne-fighting abilities.

- Shea butter and coconut oil provide deep hydration and moisture, perfect for dry skin.

4. Aromatherapeutic Benefits

Essential oils, derived from natural sources, not only benefit the skin but also engage our senses. Their aromatic profiles can have a profound impact on mood and well-being. Lavender, for example, is known for its calming properties, while citrus oils like lemon and orange can uplift and invigorate.

5. Sustainable and Eco-Friendly

Embracing natural ingredients in skincare often aligns with sustainable and eco-friendly practices. Organic farming methods, which prioritize natural ingredients, tend to have a lower environmental impact compared to conventional farming that relies heavily on synthetic chemicals. By choosing products rich in natural ingredients, you contribute to a more sustainable future for our planet.

In conclusion, the importance of natural ingredients in skincare cannot be overstated. These gifts from the Earth offer a harmonious, nutrient-rich, and gentle approach to caring for your skin. By recognizing their inherent value and embracing them in your skincare routine, you not only promote the well-being of your skin but also honor the divine wisdom of creation that provides for our needs through the bounty of the natural world.

C. Common Harmful Ingredients to Avoid

"Do not conform to the pattern of this world, but be transformed by the renewing of your mind." **(Romans 12:2, NIV).** This scriptural guidance resonates with the need to seek renewal and transformation, even in the choices we make for our skincare. To embark on a path of organic skincare and embrace natural beauty, it is essential to be aware of common harmful ingredients that can be

found in conventional skincare products. Avoiding these ingredients is a proactive step towards nurturing your skin and overall well-being.

1. Parabens

Parabens, such as methylparaben and propylparaben, are synthetic preservatives commonly used in cosmetics and skincare products to extend shelf life. However, they have been linked to disruptions in hormone balance and potential health risks. In organic skincare, natural preservatives like vitamin E or grapefruit seed extract are preferred alternatives.

2. Synthetic Fragrances

Many skincare products contain synthetic fragrances, which can be a source of skin irritation and allergies. They may also contain phthalates, which are chemicals linked to hormonal disruption. Organic skincare often uses essential oils and natural fragrance extracts for a safer and more pleasing scent.

3. Sodium Lauryl Sulfate (SLS) and Sodium Laureth Sulfate (SLES)

SLS and SLES are surfactants commonly found in foaming and cleansing products. They can strip the skin of its natural oils, leading to dryness and irritation. Organic cleansers use gentler, plant-derived alternatives to achieve cleansing without harsh effects.

4. Formaldehyde and Formaldehyde-Releasing Agents

These chemicals, found in some skincare and cosmetic products, serve as preservatives. However, they are known to be skin sensitizers and irritants. Organic skincare products avoid these chemicals in favor of safer preservation methods.

5. Petrochemicals

Ingredients like mineral oil and petroleum jelly are derived from petrochemicals. While they can create a barrier on the skin, they do not provide nourishment. Organic skincare opts for natural oils and butters, like jojoba oil and shea butter, to hydrate and protect the skin.

6. Phthalates

Phthalates are often used to enhance the flexibility and scent of products. They have been associated with endocrine disruption and potential adverse health effects. Organic skincare products are phthalate-free and prioritize safer alternatives.

7. Synthetic Colors

Artificial colors are used to achieve specific product aesthetics, but they may cause skin irritation. Organic skincare relies on natural colorants like fruit extracts and herbal infusions to add color without compromising safety.

8. Triclosan

Triclosan, an antibacterial agent, is found in some skincare and personal care products. It has raised concerns about antibiotic resistance and environmental impact. Organic skincare avoids triclosan in favor of natural antibacterial ingredients.

As you embark on your organic skincare journey, it is essential to read product labels carefully and be vigilant about these harmful ingredients. Embracing organic skincare means choosing products that not only nurture your skin but also align with your values of promoting health, sustainability, and a harmonious relationship with the natural world.

Chapter III:

Essential Tools and Ingredients

A. Tools for DIY Skincare

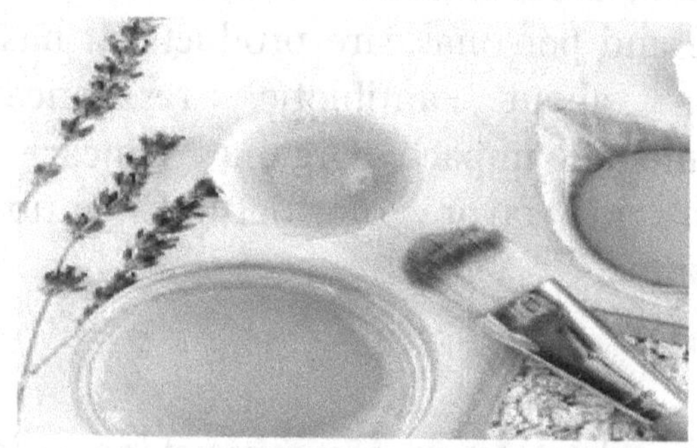

*"For every house is built by someone, but the builder of all things is God." (**Hebrews 3:4, ESV**).* Just as every house requires the right tools for construction, crafting your own skincare products necessitates a set of essential tools. These tools empower you to create with precision and care, much like the divine builder shapes the world. In this section, we will explore the tools required for your DIY skincare journey.

1. Mixing Bowls

Mixing bowls are the foundation of your DIY skincare workspace. Opt for glass or stainless steel bowls, as they are non-reactive and easy to clean. Multiple sizes come in handy for various recipes, allowing you to scale your creations as needed.

2. Measuring Utensils

Accurate measurements are crucial in skincare formulation. Invest in a set of measuring spoons and cups to ensure precise ingredient proportions. This precision helps maintain the efficacy and safety of your skincare products.

3. Whisks and Spatulas

Whisks and spatulas assist in blending and stirring ingredients thoroughly. Silicone spatulas are heat-resistant and gentle on your formulations, ensuring you can scrape every last drop from your mixing bowls.

4. Double Boiler or Heatproof Containers

Some skincare recipes involve melting ingredients, such as beeswax or shea butter. A double boiler or heatproof containers allow you to do this gently without direct heat. Alternatively, microwave-safe glass containers can serve this purpose.

5. Immersion Blender or Hand Mixer

For recipes that require emulsification, an immersion blender or hand mixer can help achieve a smooth and uniform consistency. This is especially useful when working with creams and lotions.

6. Thermometer

A thermometer is essential when precise temperature control is required. Certain ingredients, like beeswax or essential oils, have specific temperature tolerances to ensure their effectiveness.

7. Sanitization Supplies

Maintaining a clean and sterile workspace is crucial for DIY skincare. Alcohol wipes or sprays can be used to disinfect your tools and containers, preventing contamination of your products.

8. pH Strips or Meter

Checking the pH of your skincare creations is vital to ensure they are safe and suitable for your skin. pH strips or a pH meter can help you maintain the correct pH levels in your products.

9. Storage Containers

Once your skincare products are crafted, they require proper storage. Invest in a variety of glass or plastic containers with airtight lids to preserve the freshness and potency of your creations.

10. Labels and Marker

Don't underestimate the importance of labeling. Clearly mark your skincare products with their names, creation dates, and usage instructions. This ensures you can use them safely and effectively.

11. Notebook or Recipe Journal

Keeping a dedicated skincare recipe journal allows you to record your formulations, adjustments, and results. Over time, this becomes a valuable resource for refining your recipes and creating customized products.

As you gather these essential tools for DIY skincare, remember that they are the instruments through which you'll translate your vision of natural beauty into reality. Much like the builder referenced in **Hebrews 3:4,** you have the power to construct skincare products that nurture and enhance your skin while aligning with the wisdom of nature. These tools are your companions on a journey of creation and self-care, a journey that harmonizes with the divine craftsmanship of the world.

B. Essential Oils and Their Benefits

"And the Lord God made all kinds of trees grow out of the ground—trees that were pleasing to the eye and good for food." (Genesis 2:9, NIV). In these words from the book of Genesis, we find an acknowledgment of the goodness and beauty of trees and plants. Essential oils, derived from various parts of plants, capture the essence of this goodness and offer a wide array of benefits for skincare. In this section, we will explore essential oils and their remarkable contributions to DIY skincare.

1. Lavender Oil (Lavandula angustifolia)

Lavender oil is a versatile essential oil known for its calming and soothing properties. It's used to alleviate skin irritation, reduce redness, and promote relaxation. Lavender oil is often found in recipes for creams, lotions, and face masks.

2. Tea Tree Oil (Melaleuca alternifolia)

Tea tree oil is renowned for its antibacterial and antifungal properties. It's a powerful ingredient in combating acne and skin infections. When used in diluted form, it can help purify the skin without causing excessive dryness.

3. Roman Chamomile Oil (Anthemis nobilis)

Roman chamomile oil is gentle and suitable for sensitive skin. It possesses anti-inflammatory and calming properties, making it an excellent choice for soothing skin irritations, such as redness and eczema.

4. Frankincense Oil (Boswellia carterii)

Frankincense oil is treasured for its anti-aging and rejuvenating effects. It promotes the regeneration of skin cells and helps reduce the appearance of fine lines and wrinkles. It's often used in serums and anti-aging formulations.

5. Rosehip Seed Oil (Rosa canina)

While not an essential oil, rosehip seed oil is a valuable natural ingredient rich in vitamins, antioxidants, and essential fatty acids. It's known for its ability to hydrate, heal scars, and brighten the skin. It's commonly used in facial serums and moisturizers.

6. Peppermint Oil (Mentha × piperita)

Peppermint oil imparts a refreshing sensation and has a cooling effect on the skin. It's used in skincare to alleviate itching, soothe sore muscles, and invigorate the senses. It can be found in body scrubs, foot creams, and invigorating masks.

7. Geranium Oil (Pelargonium graveolens)

Geranium oil is known for its balancing properties. It helps regulate oil production, making it suitable for both dry and oily skin types. It's often used in toners and facial mists.

8. Lemon Oil (Citrus limon)

Lemon oil is bright and uplifting. It's rich in vitamin C and antioxidants, making it beneficial for brightening the complexion and promoting an even skin tone. It's used in facial cleansers and brightening serums.

9. Rose Oil (Rosa damascena)

Rose oil is a luxurious and aromatic essential oil that is cherished for its ability to hydrate and soothe the skin. It's used in high-end skincare products, including facial oils and masks, to promote a radiant complexion.

10. Eucalyptus Oil (Eucalyptus globulus)

Eucalyptus oil is known for its refreshing and invigorating scent. It's used in skincare to relieve congestion, soothe muscle aches, and promote a sense of clarity. Eucalyptus oil can be found in body washes and bath oils.

Essential oils are powerful gifts from the natural world, offering a multitude of benefits for skincare. However, it's important to use them with care, ensuring proper dilution and compatibility with your skin type. As you explore the world of DIY skincare, consider the wisdom of **Genesis 2:9** and the goodness that plants and trees offer. By incorporating essential oils into your skincare recipes, you harness the beauty and benefits of these botanical treasures, creating products that promote both outer and inner well-being.

C. Carrier Oils and Butters

"And God said, 'Let the land produce living creatures according to their kinds: the livestock, the creatures that move along the ground, and the wild animals, each according to its kind.'" **(Genesis 1:24, NIV).** In these words, we find a recognition of the diversity of life forms that the Earth has brought forth, each with unique qualities and purposes. Similarly, carrier oils and butters derived from various plants and seeds offer a diverse range of benefits for skincare. In this section, we will explore carrier oils and butters and their invaluable contributions to DIY skincare.

Carrier Oils:

1. Jojoba Oil (Simmondsia chinensis)

Jojoba oil closely resembles the natural sebum produced by our skin, making it an excellent choice for all skin types. It's a superb moisturizer and is often used in facial serums and moisturizers.

2. Coconut Oil (Cocos nucifera)

Coconut oil is rich in fatty acids and has natural antimicrobial properties. It's versatile and can be used for moisturizing the skin, removing makeup, and as a base for body scrubs.

3. Sweet Almond Oil (Prunus dulcis)

Sweet almond oil is lightweight and easily absorbed, making it suitable for all skin types. It's known for its moisturizing properties and is used in various skincare products, including massage oils and bath oils.

4. Argan Oil (Argania spinosa)

Argan oil, often referred to as ***"liquid gold,"*** is rich in vitamin E and antioxidants. It's prized for its ability to hydrate, repair, and rejuvenate the skin. It's commonly found in facial serums and hair treatments.

5. Olive Oil (Olea europaea)

Olive oil is a nourishing oil that is high in antioxidants and vitamin E. It's used for moisturizing the skin and can be included in lip balms and cuticle creams.

6. Grapeseed Oil (Vitis vinifera)

Grapeseed oil is lightweight and suitable for oily or acne-prone skin. It's often used in facial serums and can help balance skin oil production.

7. Avocado Oil (Persea americana)

Avocado oil is rich and deeply moisturizing, making it ideal for dry or mature skin. It's used in anti-aging formulations and as a base for body butters.

8. Rosehip Seed Oil (Rosa canina)

Rosehip seed oil is celebrated for its ability to promote skin regeneration and reduce the appearance of scars and fine lines. It's often found in facial oils and serums.

Butters:

1. Shea Butter (Butyrospermum parkii)

Shea butter is deeply moisturizing and rich in vitamins and fatty acids. It's used in body butters, lip balms, and creams to nourish and protect the skin.

2. Cocoa Butter (Theobroma cacao)

Cocoa butter has a rich and indulgent texture. It's known for its hydrating properties and is used in body creams, lip balms, and massage bars.

3. Mango Butter (Mangifera indica)

Mango butter is lightweight and provides excellent moisture to the skin. It's used in body and hair products to promote softness and hydration.

4. Kokum Butter (Garcinia indica)

Kokum butter is non-comedogenic and suitable for sensitive or acne-prone skin. It's often used in lip balms, creams, and lotions.

5. Avocado Butter (Persea americana)

Avocado butter is a rich and nourishing butter that contains the benefits of avocado oil. It's used in skincare products to provide deep hydration and promote skin elasticity.

6.   Cupuacu   Butter   (Theobroma grandiflorum)

Cupuacu butter is creamy and luxurious. It's used in body butters and creams for its excellent moisturizing properties and ability to improve skin texture.

These carrier oils and butters, like the diverse creatures created according to their kinds, each have their unique qualities and purposes in DIY skincare. By harnessing their natural goodness, you have the opportunity to create skincare products that honor the wisdom of nature and promote the health and radiance of your skin.

D. Herbs and Botanicals

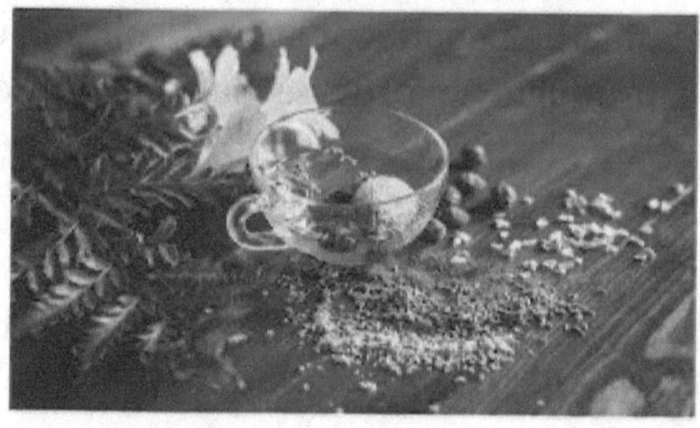

*"And God said, 'Let the land produce vegetation: seed-bearing plants and trees on the land that bear fruit with seed in it, according to their various kinds.' And it was so." **(Genesis 1:11, NIV).*** The Earth's ability to produce an abundance of vegetation, each with its unique properties and benefits, is a testament to the divine wisdom of creation. Similarly, herbs and botanicals offer a rich tapestry of natural ingredients for DIY skincare. In this section, we will explore herbs and botanicals and their valuable contributions to crafting your own skincare products.

1. Aloe Vera (Aloe barbadensis miller)

Aloe vera is a soothing and hydrating herb with anti-inflammatory properties. It's commonly used in skincare to calm irritated skin, treat sunburn, and promote healing.

2. Calendula (Calendula officinalis)

Calendula is known for its anti-inflammatory and skin-soothing properties. It's used in skincare to alleviate redness, irritation, and promote the healing of minor wounds.

3. Chamomile (Matricaria chamomilla)

Chamomile is gentle and calming, making it suitable for sensitive skin. It has anti-inflammatory and antioxidant properties and is used in skincare to reduce redness and soothe irritation.

4. Lavender (Lavandula angustifolia)

Lavender is celebrated for its soothing and relaxing properties. In skincare, it's used to calm

the skin, reduce inflammation, and promote a sense
of relaxation.

5. Rosemary (Rosmarinus officinalis)

Rosemary has antioxidant properties and is
known for stimulating blood circulation. It's used in
skincare to invigorate the skin and promote a
healthy complexion.

6. Witch Hazel (Hamamelis virginiana)

Witch hazel is a natural astringent with anti-
inflammatory properties. It's often used as a toner
to tighten the skin's pores and reduce inflammation.

7. Comfrey (Symphytum officinale)

Comfrey is rich in allantoin, a compound known
for its skin-healing properties. It's used in skincare

to promote tissue repair and soothe dry or damaged skin.

8. Green Tea (Camellia sinensis)

Green tea is rich in antioxidants and has anti-aging properties. It's used in skincare to protect the skin from environmental damage and reduce signs of aging.

9. Rose Petals (Rosa spp.)

Rose petals have astringent and anti-inflammatory properties. They are often used in skincare to soothe and tone the skin, leaving it refreshed and rejuvenated.

10. Chamomile (Matricaria chamomilla)

Oatmeal is gentle and moisturizing, making it suitable for sensitive or dry skin. It's used in skincare to soothe irritation, hydrate the skin, and promote a healthy skin barrier.

These herbs and botanicals, each with its unique characteristics and benefits, provide a wealth of options for enhancing your DIY skincare creations. By incorporating these natural ingredients into your recipes, you align with the wisdom of the Earth's vegetation and create skincare products that promote the health and radiance of your skin while honoring the divine creation described in Genesis.

Chapter IV:

Face Care Recipes

A. Cleansers and Makeup Removers

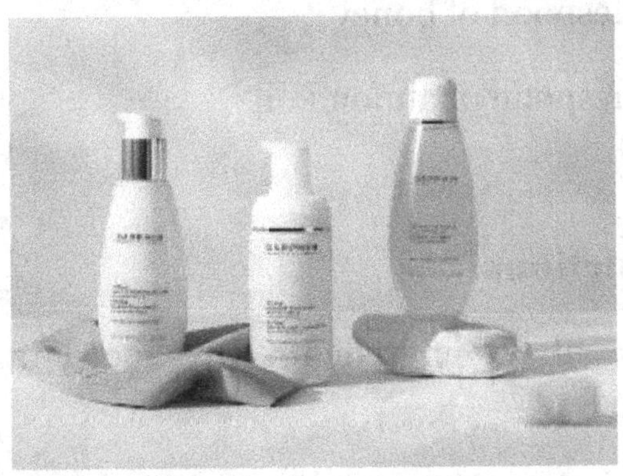

*"Wash me thoroughly from my iniquity, and cleanse me from my sin." **(Psalm 51:2, ESV).*** In this verse from the Book of Psalms, there is a recognition of the cleansing power of water and, by extension, skincare. Cleansing your face is a fundamental step in skincare, removing impurities and preparing your skin for nourishment. In this chapter, we will explore DIY recipes for cleansers and makeup removers, harnessing the goodness of natural ingredients to cleanse and purify your skin.

1. Gentle Milk Cleanser

Ingredients:

- 2 tablespoons of whole milk

- 1 tablespoon of honey

- 1 tablespoon of almond oil

Instructions:

1. Mix all the ingredients in a bowl until well combined.

2. Apply the mixture to your face using a cotton pad or your fingertips.

3. Gently massage in circular motions to remove dirt and makeup.

4. Rinse with lukewarm water and pat your face dry.

Benefits: This cleanser effectively removes makeup and impurities while providing gentle nourishment to your skin.

2. Soothing Cucumber Cleansing Water

Ingredients:

- 1 cucumber, peeled and diced

- 1/4 cup of witch hazel

Instructions:

1. Blend the diced cucumber until it becomes a smooth puree.

2. Strain the puree to extract the cucumber juice.

3. Mix the cucumber juice with witch hazel in a clean bottle.

4. Apply the cleansing water to a cotton pad and use it to wipe your face, including the eye area, to remove makeup and impurities.

Cucumber is soothing and hydrating, while witch hazel helps tone and purify the skin.

3. Oil Cleansing Blend

Ingredients:

- 2 tablespoons of castor oil

- 2 tablespoons of jojoba oil

- 1 tablespoon of sweet almond oil

- 5 drops of lavender essential oil

Instructions:

1. Combine all the oils and essential oil in a clean bottle.

2. Apply a small amount of the oil blend to your face and massage gently for a few minutes.

3. Use a warm, damp cloth to wipe away the oil, removing makeup and impurities.

Benefits: Oil cleansing effectively dissolves makeup and sebum while providing nourishment to the skin. Lavender oil adds a soothing scent.

4. Micellar Water Makeup Remover

Ingredients:

- 1/4 cup of distilled water

- 1/4 cup of witch hazel

- 1 tablespoon of vegetable glycerin

- 5 drops of chamomile essential oil

Instructions:

1. Combine all the ingredients in a clean bottle.

2. Shake well before each use.

3. Apply the micellar water to a cotton pad and gently wipe your face to remove makeup.

Benefits: Micellar water effectively lifts away makeup and dirt while chamomile oil soothes and calms the skin.

These DIY cleansers and makeup removers offer you the opportunity to cleanse your face with the purity of natural ingredients. As you use these recipes, reflect on the cleansing power they provide for your skin, and the potential for a fresh start and renewal, as expressed in Psalm 51:2.

B. Toners and Astringents

"Let your garments be always white, and let not oil be lacking on your head." (Ecclesiastes 9:8, ESV). In this verse from the Book of Ecclesiastes, there is an acknowledgment of the value of oil and anointing for personal care. Toners and astringents play a crucial role in skincare, helping to balance the skin's pH, tighten pores, and prepare it for moisturization. In this chapter, we will explore DIY recipes for toners and astringents, harnessing the goodness of natural ingredients to promote healthy and radiant skin.

1. Refreshing Rosewater Toner

Ingredients:

- 1/2 cup of rosewater

- 1/2 cup of witch hazel

- 5 drops of rose essential oil (optional)

Instructions:

1. Mix the rosewater and witch hazel in a clean bottle.

2. If desired, add the rose essential oil and shake well.

3. Apply the toner to a cotton pad and gently swipe it across your face after cleansing.

Benefits: Rosewater is soothing and hydrating, while witch hazel helps tone and balance the skin's natural oils.

2. Cooling Cucumber Astringent

Ingredients:

- 1 cucumber, peeled and diced

- 1/4 cup of distilled water

- 1/4 cup of apple cider vinegar

Instructions:

1. Blend the diced cucumber with distilled water until it becomes a smooth puree.

2. Strain the cucumber juice into a clean bottle.

3. Add the apple cider vinegar and shake well.

4. Apply the astringent to a cotton pad and gently pat it onto your face after cleansing.

Benefits: Cucumber is cooling and soothing, while apple cider vinegar acts as an astringent to help tighten pores.

3. Balancing Green Tea Toner

Ingredients:

- 1/2 cup of brewed green tea, cooled

- 1/4 cup of aloe vera gel

- 5 drops of tea tree essential oil (optional)

Instructions:

1. Mix the cooled green tea and aloe vera gel in a clean bottle.

2. If desired, add the tea tree essential oil and shake well.

3. Apply the toner to a cotton pad and gently sweep it over your face after cleansing.

Benefits: Green tea provides antioxidant protection, aloe vera soothes, and tea tree oil offers antibacterial properties.

4. Clarifying Witch Hazel Tonic

Ingredients:

- 1/2 cup of witch hazel

- 1/4 cup of distilled water

- 5 drops of lavender essential oil (optional)

Instructions:

1. Mix the witch hazel and distilled water in a clean bottle.

2. If desired, add the lavender essential oil and shake well.

3. Apply the tonic to a cotton pad and gently pat it onto your face after cleansing.

Benefits: Witch hazel is an excellent astringent, and lavender oil adds a soothing scent.

These DIY toners and astringents offer a natural and refreshing way to balance and prepare your skin. As you use these recipes, consider the wisdom of Ecclesiastes 9:8 and the value of anointing and personal care, not just for your skin but as a form of self-care and self-expression.

C. Serums and Moisturizers

"For the Lord is good; his steadfast love endures forever, and his faithfulness to all generations." **(Psalm 100:5, ESV).** In this verse from the Book of Psalms, we find a reflection of enduring love and faithfulness. Just as God's love is steadfast, your skincare routine should include serums and moisturizers that provide enduring hydration and nourishment to your skin. In this chapter, we will explore DIY recipes for serums and moisturizers, harnessing the goodness of natural ingredients to promote healthy, radiant skin.

1. Hydrating Hyaluronic Acid Serum

Ingredients:

- 1 tablespoon of aloe vera gel

- 1 tablespoon of vegetable glycerin

- 1/2 teaspoon of hyaluronic acid powder

- 2-3 drops of rosehip seed oil

Instructions:

1. In a clean bowl, mix the aloe vera gel and vegetable glycerin.

2. Add the hyaluronic acid powder and stir until it dissolves completely.

3. Stir in the rosehip seed oil.

4. Transfer the serum to a dark glass dropper bottle.

5. Apply a few drops to your face and neck after toning, then follow with a moisturizer.

Benefits: Hyaluronic acid attracts and retains moisture, while aloe vera and rosehip seed oil provide hydration and nourishment.

2. Rejuvenating Vitamin C Serum

Ingredients:

- 1/2 teaspoon of vitamin C powder (ascorbic acid)

- 1 tablespoon of distilled water

- 1 tablespoon of vegetable glycerin

- 5 drops of vitamin E oil

Instructions:

1. In a clean bowl, dissolve the vitamin C powder in distilled water.

2. Stir in the vegetable glycerin and vitamin E oil.

3. Transfer the serum to a dark glass dropper bottle.

4. Apply a few drops to your face and neck after toning, then follow with a moisturizer.

Benefits: Vitamin C is known for its brightening and antioxidant properties, while vitamin E provides added nourishment and protection.

3. Nourishing DIY Face Oil

Ingredients:

- 1 tablespoon of jojoba oil

- 1 tablespoon of rosehip seed oil

- 1 tablespoon of argan oil

- 3 drops of lavender essential oil

Instructions:

1. Mix all the oils and essential oil in a clean glass bottle.

2. Apply a few drops to your face and neck as the final step in your skincare routine.

Benefits: This face oil combines the benefits of various nourishing oils to hydrate and rejuvenate the skin.

4. Homemade Whipped Shea Butter Moisturizer

Ingredients:

- 1/2 cup of shea butter

- 2 tablespoons of coconut oil

- 1 tablespoon of sweet almond oil

- 10 drops of your favorite essential oil (e.g., lavender, rose)

Instructions:

1. In a double boiler, melt the shea butter and coconut oil until they become liquid.

2. Remove from heat and let it cool for a few minutes.

3. Stir in the sweet almond oil and essential oil of your choice.

4. Place the mixture in the refrigerator until it partially solidifies.

5. Whip the semi-solid mixture with an electric mixer until it becomes light and fluffy.

6. Transfer the whipped moisturizer to a clean jar.

Benefits: This whipped moisturizer is deeply hydrating and nourishing, leaving your skin soft and supple.

These DIY serums and moisturizers offer a natural and loving way to care for your skin, much like the enduring love and faithfulness mentioned in Psalm 100:5. As you use these recipes, consider the steadfast care you provide for your skin, nurturing it with the goodness of natural ingredients.

D. Face Masks for Different Skin Types

"And he shall be like a tree planted by the rivers of water, that bringeth forth his fruit in his season; his leaf also shall not wither, and whatsoever he doeth shall prosper." (Psalm 1:3, KJV). In this verse from the Book of Psalms, there is a beautiful metaphor comparing a flourishing tree to a life of prosperity and steadfastness. Face masks are like nourishing soil for your skin, ensuring its vitality and well-being. In this chapter, we will explore DIY face mask recipes tailored to different skin types, harnessing the goodness of natural ingredients to promote healthy and radiant skin.

1. Soothing Oatmeal and Honey Mask (For Sensitive Skin)

Ingredients:

- 2 tablespoons of ground oats

- 1 tablespoon of honey

- 1 tablespoon of plain yogurt

Instructions:

1. Mix the ground oats, honey, and yogurt in a bowl to form a paste.

2. Apply the mixture to your clean face and leave it on for 15-20 minutes.

3. Rinse off with lukewarm water and pat your skin dry.

Benefits: This mask soothes and calms sensitive skin, reducing redness and irritation.

2. Brightening Turmeric and Yogurt Mask (For Dull Skin)

Ingredients:

- 1/2 teaspoon of turmeric powder

- 2 tablespoons of plain yogurt

- 1 teaspoon of honey

Instructions:

1. Mix the turmeric powder, yogurt, and honey in a bowl until well combined.

2. Apply the mixture to your clean face and leave it on for 10-15 minutes.

3. Rinse off with lukewarm water and pat your skin dry.

Benefits: Turmeric brightens the complexion, yogurt exfoliates, and honey hydrates, leaving your skin radiant.

3. Hydrating Avocado and Banana Mask (For Dry Skin)

Ingredients:

- 1/2 ripe avocado

- 1/2 ripe banana

- 1 tablespoon of honey

Instructions:

1. Mash the avocado and banana together in a bowl.

2. Stir in the honey to create a smooth paste.

3. Apply the mixture to your clean face and leave it on for 15-20 minutes.

4. Rinse off with lukewarm water and pat your skin dry.

Benefits: This mask provides deep hydration for dry skin, leaving it soft and nourished.

4. Clarifying Clay and Tea Tree Mask (For Oily or Acne-Prone Skin)

Ingredients:

- 1 tablespoon of green clay

- 1-2 drops of tea tree essential oil

- 1 tablespoon of water (or more as needed)

Instructions:

1. In a bowl, mix the green clay, tea tree essential oil, and enough water to create a thick paste.

2. Apply the clay mask to your clean face, avoiding the eye area.

3. Leave it on until it dries (about 10-15 minutes).

4. Rinse off with lukewarm water and pat your skin dry.

Benefits: Green clay helps absorb excess oil and impurities, while tea tree oil has antibacterial properties to combat acne.

These DIY face masks, tailored to different skin types, are like the nourishing soil that sustains a flourishing tree. As you apply these masks to your skin, consider the prosperity and steadfastness of the tree mentioned in Psalm 1:3 and how these masks promote the health and vitality of your skin.

Chapter V:

Body Care Recipes

A. Homemade Body Washes and Scrubs

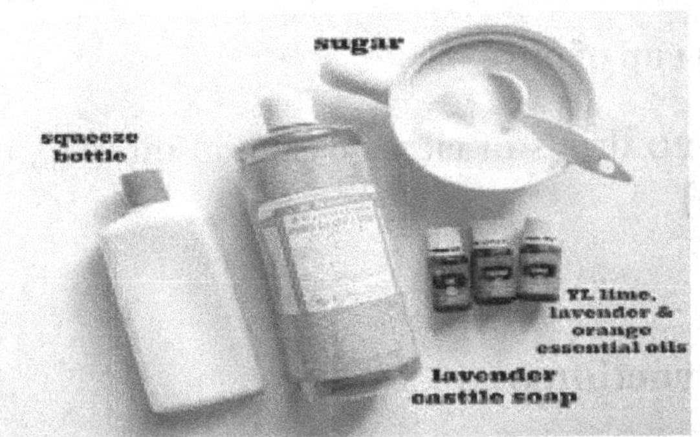

"For we are God's handiwork, created in Christ Jesus to do good works, which God prepared in advance for us to do." **(Ephesians 2:10, NIV).** In this verse from the Book of Ephesians, there is a recognition of our divine creation and purpose. Caring for your body is an act of self-care and self-love, much like how God's handiwork deserves to be nurtured. In this chapter, we will explore DIY recipes for body washes and scrubs, using natural ingredients to cleanse and pamper your body.

1. Energizing Citrus Body Wash

Ingredients:

- 1/2 cup of liquid castile soap

- 1/4 cup of honey

- 1/4 cup of olive oil

- 15-20 drops of citrus essential oil (e.g., orange, lemon)

Instructions:

1. Mix the liquid castile soap, honey, and olive oil in a bottle.

2. Add the citrus essential oil and shake well.

3. Use the body wash with a loofah or washcloth to cleanse your body in the shower.

Benefits: This invigorating body wash cleanses and uplifts your spirits with the refreshing scent of citrus.

2. Exfoliating Coffee Scrub

Ingredients:

- 1/2 cup of ground coffee

- 1/4 cup of coconut oil

- 1/4 cup of brown sugar

Instructions:

1. Mix the ground coffee, coconut oil, and brown sugar in a bowl.

2. In the shower, apply the scrub to damp skin in circular motions, focusing on rough areas.

3. Rinse thoroughly and pat your skin dry.

Benefits: This scrub exfoliates and smooths your skin while the caffeine in coffee can temporarily reduce the appearance of cellulite.

3. Calming Lavender Body Wash

Ingredients:

- 1/2 cup of liquid castile soap

- 1/4 cup of aloe vera gel

- 1/4 cup of sweet almond oil

- 10-15 drops of lavender essential oil

Instructions:

1. Mix the liquid castile soap, aloe vera gel, and sweet almond oil in a bottle.

2. Add the lavender essential oil and shake well.

3. Use the body wash to cleanse and relax in the shower.

Benefits: Lavender's calming properties make this body wash ideal for winding down after a long day.

4. Sugar and Honey Body Scrub

Ingredients:

- 1 cup of granulated sugar

- 1/4 cup of honey

- 1/4 cup of coconut oil

- 1 teaspoon of vanilla extract (optional)

Instructions:

1. Mix the granulated sugar, honey, coconut oil, and vanilla extract (if using) in a bowl.

2. In the shower, apply the scrub to damp skin in gentle circular motions.

3. Rinse thoroughly and pat your skin dry.

Benefits: This sweet and luxurious scrub exfoliates and moisturizes your skin, leaving it soft and radiant.

These DIY body washes and scrubs are like acts of self-care and self-love, much like how we are God's handiwork, deserving of care and nurturing as mentioned in Ephesians 2:10. As you use these recipes, consider the loving care you provide for your body, nourishing it with the goodness of natural ingredients.

B. Natural Deodorants

"Therefore, as God's chosen people, holy and dearly loved, clothe yourselves with compassion, kindness, humility, gentleness and patience." **(Colossians 3:12, NIV).** In this verse from the Book of Colossians, there is an exhortation to clothe ourselves with virtues like compassion and kindness. Just as we clothe ourselves with these virtues, we also clothe our bodies with deodorants to care for them. In this chapter, we will explore DIY recipes for natural deodorants, using

ingredients that are gentle on your skin and effective in keeping you fresh.

1. Baking Soda and Coconut Oil Deodorant

Ingredients:

- 1/4 cup of baking soda

- 1/4 cup of cornstarch

- 6 tablespoons of coconut oil

- 10-15 drops of your favorite essential oil (e.g., lavender, tea tree)

Instructions:

1. In a bowl, mix the baking soda and cornstarch.

2. Add the coconut oil and essential oil, then stir until it forms a paste.

3. Transfer the mixture to an empty deodorant container or a small jar.

4. Allow it to cool and solidify, then apply a small amount to your underarms as needed.

Benefits: Baking soda neutralizes odors, cornstarch helps absorb moisture, and coconut oil nourishes the skin.

2. Shea Butter and Arrowroot Powder Deodorant

Ingredients:

- 3 tablespoons of shea butter

- 3 tablespoons of arrowroot powder

- 2 tablespoons of baking soda

- 10-15 drops of your favorite essential oil (e.g., eucalyptus, lemongrass)

Instructions:

1. Melt the shea butter in a double boiler.

2. Remove from heat and stir in the arrowroot powder and baking soda.

3. Add the essential oil and mix well.

4. Pour the mixture into an empty deodorant container or a small jar.

5. Allow it to cool and solidify, then apply a small amount to your underarms as needed.

Benefits: Shea butter provides moisture, arrowroot powder absorbs sweat, and baking soda neutralizes odors.

3. Coconut Oil and Beeswax Deodorant Stick

Ingredients:

- 3 tablespoons of coconut oil

- 1 tablespoon of beeswax pellets

- 2 tablespoons of baking soda

- 2 tablespoons of cornstarch

- 10-15 drops of your favorite essential oil (e.g., lavender, lemon)

Instructions:

1. In a double boiler, melt the coconut oil and beeswax pellets.

2. Remove from heat and stir in the baking soda, cornstarch, and essential oil.

3. Pour the mixture into an empty deodorant container and allow it to cool and solidify.

4. Apply to your underarms as needed.

Benefits: Beeswax provides a solid texture, coconut oil moisturizes, and essential oils add fragrance.

4. Aloe Vera and Witch Hazel Spray Deodorant

Ingredients:

- 1/4 cup of aloe vera gel

- 1/4 cup of witch hazel

- 10-15 drops of tea tree essential oil

- 10-15 drops of lavender essential oil

Instructions:

1. Mix the aloe vera gel, witch hazel, and essential oils in a spray bottle.

2. Shake well before each use.

3. Spritz the deodorant onto your underarms and allow it to dry.

Benefits: Aloe vera soothes, witch hazel tones, and tea tree oil offers antibacterial properties.

These DIY natural deodorants are like acts of compassion and kindness toward your body, as mentioned in Colossians 3:12. As you use these recipes, consider the care and gentleness you provide for your body, choosing ingredients that are both effective and nurturing.

C. Body Lotions and Creams

"I praise you because I am fearfully and wonderfully made; your works are wonderful, I know that full well." **(Psalm 139:14, NIV).** In this verse from the Book of Psalms, there is a recognition of the wonder of our creation. Just as we are fearfully and wonderfully made, our bodies deserve to be pampered with lotions and creams that celebrate their uniqueness. In this chapter, we will explore DIY recipes for body lotions and creams, using natural ingredients to nourish and hydrate your skin.

1. Luxurious Shea Butter Body Lotion

Ingredients:

- 1/2 cup of shea butter

- 1/4 cup of coconut oil

- 1/4 cup of almond oil

- 10-15 drops of your favorite essential oil (e.g., lavender, rose)

Instructions:

1. In a double boiler, melt the shea butter and coconut oil.

2. Remove from heat and stir in the almond oil and essential oil.

3. Allow the mixture to cool for a few minutes, then place it in the refrigerator until it partially solidifies.

4. Whip the semi-solid mixture with an electric mixer until it becomes light and fluffy.

5. Transfer the whipped lotion to a clean jar.

Benefits: This shea butter lotion is deeply hydrating and leaves your skin soft and supple.

2. Nourishing Cocoa Butter Body Cream

Ingredients:

- 1/2 cup of cocoa butter

- 1/4 cup of coconut oil

- 1/4 cup of jojoba oil

- 10-15 drops of vanilla essential oil (optional)

Instructions:

1. In a double boiler, melt the cocoa butter and coconut oil.

2. Remove from heat and stir in the jojoba oil and vanilla essential oil (if using).

3. Allow the mixture to cool for a few minutes, then place it in the refrigerator until it partially solidifies.

4. Whip the semi-solid mixture with an electric mixer until it becomes light and fluffy.

5. Transfer the whipped cream to a clean jar.

Benefits: This cocoa butter cream is indulgent and deeply moisturizing, leaving your skin with a subtle cocoa fragrance.

3. Soothing Aloe Vera and Calendula Lotion

Ingredients:

- 1/2 cup of aloe vera gel

- 1/4 cup of calendula-infused oil

- 1/4 cup of beeswax pellets

- 10-15 drops of chamomile essential oil

Instructions:

1. In a double boiler, melt the beeswax pellets and calendula-infused oil.

2. Remove from heat and stir in the aloe vera gel and chamomile essential oil.

3. Allow the mixture to cool for a few minutes, then place it in the refrigerator until it partially solidifies.

4. Whip the semi-solid mixture with an electric mixer until it becomes light and creamy.

5. Transfer the soothing lotion to a clean jar.

Benefits: Aloe vera and calendula are soothing for the skin, making this lotion ideal for sensitive or irritated skin.

4. Cooling Peppermint and Eucalyptus Lotion

Ingredients:

- 1/2 cup of coconut oil

- 1/4 cup of almond oil

- 10-15 drops of peppermint essential oil

- 10-15 drops of eucalyptus essential oil

Instructions:

1. In a bowl, mix the coconut oil, almond oil, peppermint essential oil, and eucalyptus essential oil.

2. Whip the mixture with an electric mixer until it becomes light and fluffy.

3. Transfer the cooling lotion to a clean jar.

Benefits: Peppermint and eucalyptus provide a refreshing and cooling sensation, making this lotion perfect for hot weather.

These DIY body lotions and creams celebrate the uniqueness of your body, just as you are fearfully and wonderfully made, as mentioned in ***Psalm 139:14.*** As you use these recipes, consider the wonderful work you do in caring for your skin, nurturing it with the goodness of natural ingredients.

D. Sunscreen and After-Sun Care

 In this verse from the Book of Psalms, there is a plea for protection and a call for rejoicing in it. Protecting your skin from the sun's harmful rays is an act of self-care and self-love. In this chapter, we will explore DIY recipes for sunscreen and after-sun care, using natural ingredients to shield and soothe your skin.

1. Homemade Natural Sunscreen

Ingredients:

- 1/4 cup of coconut oil

- 1/4 cup of shea butter

- 1/4 cup of beeswax pellets

- 2 tablespoons of zinc oxide powder (non-nano)

- 1 teaspoon of carrot seed oil

- 10-15 drops of lavender essential oil (optional)

Instructions:

1. In a double boiler, melt the coconut oil, shea butter, and beeswax pellets.

2. Remove from heat and stir in the zinc oxide powder, carrot seed oil, and lavender essential oil (if using).

3. Pour the mixture into a clean container, such as a tin or a small jar.

4. Allow it to cool and solidify.

Benefits: This natural sunscreen provides broad-spectrum protection with zinc oxide and nourishing ingredients like coconut oil and shea butter.

2. Soothing Aloe Vera and Lavender After-Sun Spray

Ingredients:

- 1/2 cup of aloe vera gel

- 1/4 cup of distilled water

- 10-15 drops of lavender essential oil

Instructions:

1. Mix the aloe vera gel, distilled water, and lavender essential oil in a spray bottle.

2. Shake well before each use.

3. Spritz the soothing after-sun spray onto sun-exposed skin for instant relief.

Benefits: Aloe vera calms and hydrates sunburned skin, while lavender essential oil provides a soothing scent.

3. Cooling Cucumber and Mint After-Sun Lotion

Ingredients:

- 1/2 cucumber, peeled and diced

- 1/4 cup of coconut oil

- 1/4 cup of almond oil

- 10-15 drops of peppermint essential oil

Instructions:

1. Blend the diced cucumber until it becomes a smooth puree.

2. In a bowl, mix the cucumber puree, coconut oil, almond oil, and peppermint essential oil.

3. Transfer the mixture to a clean container.

4. Store it in the refrigerator for a cooling effect.

5. Apply the after-sun lotion to sun-exposed skin for relief.

Benefits: Cucumber soothes and hydrates, while peppermint provides a refreshing sensation.

4. Repairing Coconut Oil and Vitamin E Lip Balm

Ingredients:

- 2 tablespoons of coconut oil

- 1 tablespoon of beeswax pellets

- 1/2 teaspoon of vitamin E oil

- 10-15 drops of your favorite essential oil (e.g., peppermint, orange)

Instructions:

1. In a double boiler, melt the coconut oil and beeswax pellets.

2. Remove from heat and stir in the vitamin E oil and essential oil.

3. Pour the mixture into lip balm containers.

4. Allow it to cool and solidify.

Benefits: This lip balm soothes and nourishes dry, sun-exposed lips.

These DIY sunscreen and after-sun care recipes offer protection and relief, much like the plea for protection and rejoicing in it mentioned in **Psalm 5:11.** As you use these recipes, consider the care and protection you provide for your skin, shielding it from the sun's rays and soothing it with the goodness of natural ingredients.

Chapter VI:

Hair Care Recipes

A. Shampoos and Conditioners

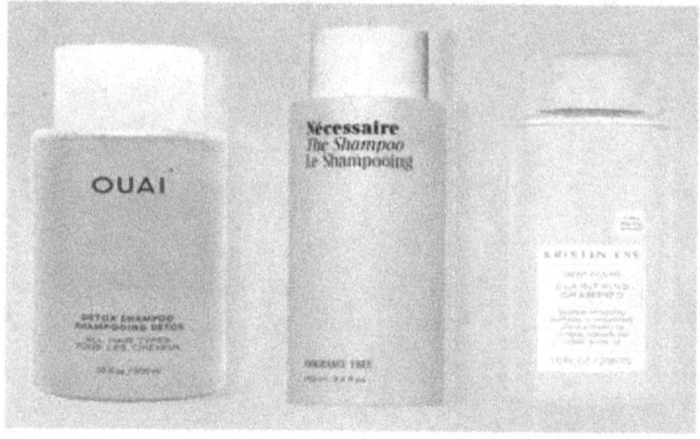

"But the very hairs of your head are all numbered. Fear not therefore: ye are of more value than many sparrows." **(Luke 12:7, KJV).** In this verse from the Book of Luke, there is a reminder of our intrinsic value. Just as God cares for us down to the very hairs of our head, we should care for our hair with love and attention. In this chapter, we will explore DIY recipes for shampoos and conditioners, using natural ingredients to cleanse and nourish your hair.

1. Nourishing Coconut Milk Shampoo

Ingredients:

- 1/2 cup of coconut milk

- 1/4 cup of liquid castile soap

- 1 tablespoon of almond oil

- 10-15 drops of your favorite essential oil (e.g., lavender, rosemary)

Instructions:

1. In a bowl, mix the coconut milk, liquid castile soap, almond oil, and essential oil.

2. Transfer the shampoo to an empty bottle.

3. Shake well before each use.

4. Use as you would regular shampoo.

Benefits: Coconut milk is hydrating, castile soap cleanses gently, and essential oils add fragrance and hair-nourishing properties.

2. Revitalizing Apple Cider Vinegar Conditioner

Ingredients:

- 1/2 cup of apple cider vinegar

- 1/2 cup of water

- 10-15 drops of lavender essential oil (optional)

Instructions:

1. Mix the apple cider vinegar, water, and lavender essential oil (if using) in an empty bottle.

2. Shake well before each use.

3. After shampooing, pour the conditioner over your hair, focusing on the ends.

4. Leave it on for a few minutes, then rinse thoroughly.

Benefits: Apple cider vinegar balances the pH of your hair, leaving it soft and shiny.

3. Strengthening Egg and Honey Shampoo

Ingredients:

- 2 eggs

- 2 tablespoons of honey

- 1 tablespoon of olive oil

Instructions:

1. In a bowl, beat the eggs and mix in the honey and olive oil until well combined.

2. Wet your hair, then apply the mixture to your scalp and hair.

3. Massage gently for a few minutes.

4. Rinse with cool water (hot water may cook the eggs) and follow with a mild conditioner if needed.

Benefits: Eggs provide protein for hair strength, honey adds moisture, and olive oil nourishes.

4. Hydrating Avocado and Yogurt Conditioner

Ingredients:

- 1 ripe avocado

- 1/2 cup of plain yogurt

- 1 tablespoon of honey

Instructions:

1. Mash the avocado and mix it with the yogurt and honey until smooth.

2. After shampooing, apply the mixture to your hair, focusing on the ends.

3. Leave it on for 15-20 minutes.

4. Rinse thoroughly with cool water.

Benefits: Avocado and yogurt moisturize and condition your hair, leaving it soft and manageable.

These DIY shampoos and conditioners celebrate the value of your hair, just as God values us down to the very hairs of our head, as mentioned in Luke 12:7. As you use these recipes, consider the love and attention you provide for your hair, nurturing it with the goodness of natural ingredients.

B. Scalp Treatments

"He makes me lie down in green pastures, he leads me beside quiet waters, he refreshes my soul." (Psalm 23:2-3, NIV). In this excerpt from *Psalm 23,* there is a sense of refreshment and rejuvenation by quiet waters. Just as our souls are refreshed, our scalps deserve to be rejuvenated and cared for. In this chapter, we will explore DIY recipes for scalp treatments, using natural ingredients to nourish and revitalize your scalp.

1. Moisturizing Coconut and Aloe Vera Scalp Treatment

Ingredients:

- 1/4 cup of coconut oil

- 1/4 cup of aloe vera gel

- 10-15 drops of tea tree essential oil

Instructions:

1. In a bowl, mix the coconut oil, aloe vera gel, and tea tree essential oil.

2. Part your hair and apply the treatment directly to your scalp.

3. Massage gently for a few minutes to distribute the mixture.

4. Leave it on for at least 30 minutes or overnight.

5. Shampoo and condition your hair as usual.

Benefits: Coconut oil moisturizes, aloe vera soothes, and tea tree oil has antibacterial properties to promote a healthy scalp.

2. Exfoliating Brown Sugar and Olive Oil Scalp Scrub

Ingredients:

- 2 tablespoons of brown sugar

- 2 tablespoons of olive oil

- 5-10 drops of rosemary essential oil

Instructions:

1. Mix the brown sugar, olive oil, and rosemary essential oil in a bowl.

2. Part your hair and apply the scrub directly to your scalp.

3. Gently massage in circular motions to exfoliate the scalp.

4. Leave it on for 10-15 minutes.

5. Shampoo and condition your hair as usual.

Benefits: Brown sugar exfoliates, olive oil moisturizes, and rosemary essential oil stimulates the scalp.

3. Revitalizing Green Tea and Lemon Scalp Rinse

Ingredients:

- 1 cup of brewed green tea (cooled)

- Juice of 1 lemon

- 5-10 drops of peppermint essential oil

Instructions:

1. Mix the brewed green tea, lemon juice, and peppermint essential oil in a bowl.

2. After shampooing and conditioning, pour the rinse over your hair and scalp.

3. Massage gently for a few minutes.

4. Rinse with cool water.

Benefits: Green tea contains antioxidants, lemon juice clarifies, and peppermint essential oil refreshes the scalp.

4. Strengthening Egg and Yogurt Scalp Mask

Ingredients:

- 1 egg

- 1/4 cup of plain yogurt

- 1 tablespoon of honey

Instructions:

1. In a bowl, beat the egg and mix in the yogurt and honey until well combined.

2. Part your hair and apply the mask directly to your scalp.

3. Massage gently for a few minutes.

4. Leave it on for 20-30 minutes.

5. Shampoo and condition your hair as usual.

Benefits: Eggs provide protein for hair strength, yogurt soothes, and honey adds moisture.

These DIY scalp treatments offer refreshment and rejuvenation for your scalp, much like the sense of renewal by quiet waters mentioned in *Psalm 23:2-3.* As you use these recipes, consider the care and rejuvenation you provide for your scalp, nurturing it with the goodness of natural ingredients.

C. Hair Masks and Serums

"Your beauty should not come from outward adornment, such as elaborate hairstyles and the wearing of gold jewelry or fine clothes. Rather, it should be that of your inner self, the unfading beauty of a gentle and quiet spirit, which is of great worth in God's sight." (1 Peter 3:3-4, NIV).

In this passage from *1 Peter*, there is a reflection on inner beauty and its great worth. While inner beauty is paramount, caring for your hair can be an expression of self-care and self-respect. In this chapter, we will explore DIY recipes for hair masks and serums, using natural ingredients to enhance the health and beauty of your hair.

1. Deep Conditioning Avocado and Olive Oil Hair Mask

Ingredients:

- 1 ripe avocado

- 2 tablespoons of olive oil

- 1 tablespoon of honey

- 1 egg yolk

Instructions:

1. Mash the avocado and mix it with olive oil, honey, and egg yolk until it forms a smooth paste.

2. Apply the mask to clean, damp hair, focusing on the ends.

3. Cover your hair with a shower cap or towel and leave it on for 30-45 minutes.

4. Rinse thoroughly and shampoo and condition as usual.

Benefits: Avocado provides deep hydration, olive oil nourishes, honey adds moisture, and egg yolk strengthens hair.

2. Repairing Coconut Milk and Argan Oil Hair Mask

Ingredients:

- 1/2 cup of coconut milk

- 2 tablespoons of argan oil

- 10-15 drops of lavender essential oil

Instructions:

1. In a bowl, mix the coconut milk, argan oil, and lavender essential oil.

2. Apply the mask to clean, damp hair, working it through from roots to ends.

3. Leave it on for 20-30 minutes.

4. Rinse thoroughly and shampoo and condition as usual.

Benefits: Coconut milk provides moisture, argan oil repairs, and lavender essential oil adds a calming scent.

3. Hair Growth Serum with Rosemary and Castor Oil

Ingredients:

- 2 tablespoons of castor oil

- 1 tablespoon of jojoba oil

- 5-10 drops of rosemary essential oil

Instructions:

1. Mix the castor oil, jojoba oil, and rosemary essential oil in a small bottle.

2. Before bed, apply a few drops of the serum to your scalp and massage it in.

3. Leave it on overnight.

4. In the morning, shampoo and condition as usual.

Benefits: Castor oil promotes hair growth, jojoba oil moisturizes, and rosemary essential oil stimulates the scalp.

4. Strengthening Banana and Honey Hair Mask

Ingredients:

- 1 ripe banana

- 2 tablespoons of honey

- 1 tablespoon of coconut oil

Instructions:

1. Mash the banana and mix it with honey and coconut oil until it forms a smooth paste.

2. Apply the mask to clean, damp hair, focusing on the lengths and ends.

3. Leave it on for 20-30 minutes.

4. Rinse thoroughly and shampoo and condition as usual.

Benefits: Banana strengthens hair, honey adds moisture, and coconut oil nourishes.

These DIY hair masks and serums are an expression of self-care and self-respect for your hair, echoing the idea of inner beauty and its great worth mentioned in *1 Peter 3:3-4*. As you use these recipes, consider the care and respect you provide for your hair, enhancing its health and beauty with the goodness of natural ingredients.

D. Tips for Healthy Hair

In this chapter, we will explore essential tips and practices for maintaining healthy and beautiful hair. These tips are like wisdom for your locks, helping you care for your hair with love and attention.

1. Balanced Diet and Hydration

Just as our bodies need nourishment to thrive, our hair benefits from a balanced diet rich in vitamins, minerals, and protein. Incorporate foods like fruits, vegetables, lean proteins, and whole grains into your meals. Stay hydrated by drinking plenty of water, which helps keep your hair hydrated from the inside out.

2. Gentle Hair Care

Treat your hair with gentleness. Avoid harsh brushing, particularly when your hair is wet, as it can cause breakage. Use a wide-toothed comb to detangle, starting at the tips and working your way up. Choose hair accessories that are gentle on your hair, like scrunchies instead of tight elastics.

3. Regular Trims

Don't skip regular trims. Trimming your hair every 6-8 weeks helps prevent split ends and promotes healthier, shinier hair. Even if you're growing your hair out, these small trims are essential for maintaining its overall health.

4. Protect from Heat

Heat styling tools like hairdryers, straighteners, and curling irons can damage your hair over time. Use them sparingly and always apply a heat protectant spray before styling. Consider air-drying your hair whenever possible to minimize heat exposure.

5. Natural Hair Care Products

Opt for natural and organic hair care products free from harsh chemicals and sulfates. These products are gentler on your hair and scalp, helping maintain their natural balance.

6. Scalp Massage

Regular scalp massages stimulate blood circulation, which can promote hair growth and overall scalp health. Use your fingertips to gently massage your scalp for a few minutes each day, or incorporate essential oils for added benefits.

7. Protect from UV Rays

Just as you protect your skin from the sun, your hair needs protection too. Wear a wide-brimmed hat or use hair products with built-in UV protection to shield your hair from sun damage.

8. Choose the Right Shampoo and Conditioner

Select shampoos and conditioners that match your hair type. Whether you have oily, dry, curly, or straight hair, using products tailored to your needs ensures your hair gets the right care.

9. Avoid Overwashing

Overwashing can strip your hair of its natural oils, leaving it dry and brittle. Wash your hair as needed based on your hair type and lifestyle. Consider using a dry shampoo between washes to refresh your hair.

10. Manage Stress

High levels of stress can negatively impact your hair's health. Practice stress-management techniques like meditation, yoga, or deep breathing exercises to keep both your mind and hair in a healthier state.

These tips for healthy hair are like a guide to maintaining its beauty and vitality. As you incorporate these practices into your hair care routine, remember that nurturing your hair is an act of self-care and self-respect, reflecting the inner beauty mentioned in *1 Peter 3:3-4.*

Chapter VII:

Hand and Foot Care Recipes

A. Homemade Hand Creams and Scrubs

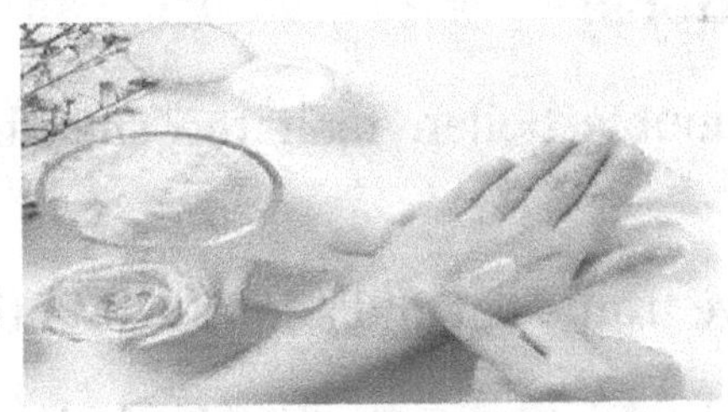

In this chapter, we will explore DIY recipes for hand creams and scrubs, using natural ingredients to pamper and rejuvenate your hands, which work tirelessly every day. Additionally, we will discuss recipes for foot care, as our feet carry us through life's journey and deserve attention and care.

1. Nourishing Shea Butter Hand Cream

Ingredients:

- 1/4 cup of shea butter

- 1/4 cup of coconut oil

- 10-15 drops of your favorite essential oil (e.g., lavender, chamomile)

Instructions:

1. In a double boiler, melt the shea butter and coconut oil.

2. Remove from heat and add the essential oil.

3. Allow the mixture to cool and solidify.

4. Whip the semi-solid mixture until it becomes creamy.

5. Transfer the hand cream to a clean jar.

Benefits: Shea butter is deeply moisturizing, and essential oils add a delightful fragrance.

2. Exfoliating Lemon and Sugar Hand Scrub

Ingredients:

- 1/2 cup of granulated sugar

- Juice of 1 lemon

- 2 tablespoons of olive oil

Instructions:

1. Mix the granulated sugar, lemon juice, and olive oil in a bowl.

2. Apply the scrub to your hands and massage gently for a few minutes.

3. Rinse with warm water and pat dry.

Benefits: Sugar exfoliates, lemon brightens, and olive oil moisturizes.

3. Soothing Lavender and Oatmeal Hand Cream

Ingredients:

- 1/4 cup of oats (finely ground)

- 1/4 cup of coconut oil

- 10-15 drops of lavender essential oil

Instructions:

1. In a blender, grind the oats into a fine powder.

2. In a bowl, mix the ground oats, coconut oil, and lavender essential oil.

3. Allow the mixture to cool and solidify.

4. Whip the semi-solid mixture until it becomes creamy.

5. Transfer the hand cream to a clean jar.

Benefits: Oats soothe irritated skin, coconut oil hydrates, and lavender essential oil provides a calming scent.

4. Peppermint and Epsom Salt Foot Scrub

Ingredients:

- 1/2 cup of Epsom salt

- 2 tablespoons of coconut oil

- 10-15 drops of peppermint essential oil

Instructions:

1. Mix the Epsom salt, coconut oil, and peppermint essential oil in a bowl.

2. Gently massage the scrub onto your feet, paying attention to rough areas.

3. Rinse with warm water and pat dry.

Benefits: Epsom salt exfoliates, coconut oil moisturizes, and peppermint essential oil refreshes tired feet.

These DIY hand creams and scrubs, along with the foot scrub, are like acts of gratitude and care for your hardworking hands and feet. As you use these recipes, remember the importance of self-care and the rejuvenation it brings to both body and spirit.

B. Nail and Cuticle Care

In this section, we will explore DIY recipes for nail and cuticle care, because healthy nails and cuticles are essential components of well-groomed hands.

1. Nourishing Cuticle Oil

Ingredients:

- 2 tablespoons of jojoba oil

- 5-10 drops of vitamin E oil

- 5-10 drops of lavender essential oil

Instructions:

1. In a small bottle, combine the jojoba oil, vitamin E oil, and lavender essential oil.

2. Shake well to mix the oils thoroughly.

3. Apply a drop or two of the cuticle oil to each nail and massage gently.

4. Use daily to keep your cuticles soft and hydrated.

Benefits: Jojoba oil hydrates, vitamin E oil promotes nail health, and lavender essential oil provides a pleasant aroma.

2. DIY Nail Strengthening Soak

Ingredients:

- 1 tablespoon of olive oil

- Juice of half a lemon

- 1/4 cup of warm water

Instructions:

1. Mix the olive oil and lemon juice in a small bowl.

2. Soak your nails in the warm water for a few minutes to soften them.

3. Apply the olive oil and lemon juice mixture to your nails and cuticles.

4. Massage gently and leave it on for 10-15 minutes.

5. Rinse with warm water and pat dry.

Benefits: Olive oil nourishes nails, lemon juice brightens, and the warm soak softens cuticles.

3. Homemade Nail and Cuticle Cream

Ingredients:

- 2 tablespoons of shea butter

- 1 tablespoon of beeswax pellets

- 1 tablespoon of almond oil

- 5-10 drops of your favorite essential oil (e.g., rosemary, tea tree)

Instructions:

1. In a double boiler, melt the shea butter and beeswax pellets.

2. Remove from heat and stir in the almond oil and essential oil.

3. Pour the mixture into a clean container, such as a tin or a small jar.

4. Allow it to cool and solidify.

5. Apply the cream to your nails and cuticles as needed.

Benefits: Shea butter moisturizes, beeswax protects, and essential oils add a pleasant scent while promoting nail health.

4. Strengthening Biotin-Rich Smoothie

Ingredients:

- 1 banana

- 1/2 cup of strawberries

- 1/2 cup of spinach

- 1/2 cup of almond milk

- 1 tablespoon of flaxseeds

- 1 biotin supplement (crushed and mixed in)

Instructions:

1. Blend all the ingredients until you have a smoothie.

2. Consume this biotin-rich smoothie daily to promote nail strength and overall health.

Benefits: Biotin strengthens nails, and the other ingredients provide essential vitamins and minerals.

These DIY nail and cuticle care recipes help you maintain well-groomed nails and healthy cuticles.

As you practice these nail-care routines, remember that taking care of your nails is a form of self-expression and self-care, enhancing the overall beauty and health of your hands.

C. Foot Soaks and Balms

Your feet, which carry you through life's journey, deserve special attention and care. In this section, we will explore DIY recipes for foot soaks and balms to pamper and rejuvenate your hardworking feet.

1. Relaxing Epsom Salt Foot Soak

Ingredients:

- 1/2 cup of Epsom salt

- 1/4 cup of baking soda

- 10-15 drops of lavender essential oil

Instructions:

1. Fill a basin with warm water.

2. Add the Epsom salt, baking soda, and lavender essential oil.

3. Stir to dissolve the salts and oil.

4. Soak your feet for 15-20 minutes, allowing the mixture to relax and refresh your feet.

Benefits: Epsom salt relaxes muscles, baking soda exfoliates, and lavender essential oil provides a calming aroma.

2. Peppermint and Tea Tree Oil Foot Balm

Ingredients:

- 1/4 cup of shea butter

- 1/4 cup of coconut oil

- 10-15 drops of peppermint essential oil

- 5-10 drops of tea tree essential oil

Instructions:

1. In a double boiler, melt the shea butter and coconut oil.

2. Remove from heat and add the peppermint and tea tree essential oils.

3. Allow the mixture to cool and solidify.

4. Whip the semi-solid mixture until it becomes creamy.

5. Apply the balm to your feet, especially dry or rough areas.

Benefits: Shea butter and coconut oil moisturize, while peppermint and tea tree essential oils provide a refreshing and antifungal effect.

3. Invigorating Lemon and Sea Salt Foot Scrub

Ingredients:

- Zest of 1 lemon

- Juice of 1 lemon

- 1/2 cup of sea salt

- 2 tablespoons of olive oil

Instructions:

1. Mix the lemon zest, lemon juice, sea salt, and olive oil in a bowl.

2. Apply the scrub to your feet and massage gently for a few minutes, paying attention to rough areas.

3. Rinse with warm water and pat dry.

Benefits: Lemon brightens and exfoliates, sea salt exfoliates, and olive oil moisturizes.

4. Soothing Aloe Vera and Lavender Foot Spray

Ingredients:

- 1/2 cup of aloe vera gel

- 1/4 cup of distilled water

- 10-15 drops of lavender essential oil

Instructions:

1. Mix the aloe vera gel, distilled water, and lavender essential oil in a spray bottle.

2. Shake well before each use.

3. Spritz the soothing foot spray on tired feet for instant relief.

Benefits: Aloe vera soothes and hydrates, and lavender essential oil provides a calming scent.

These DIY foot soaks and balms are like acts of gratitude and care for your hardworking feet. As you use these recipes, remember the importance of self-care and the rejuvenation it brings to both body and spirit, especially for your feet that carry you through life's journey.

Chapter VIII:

Specialized Skincare Recipes

A. Anti-Aging Formulas

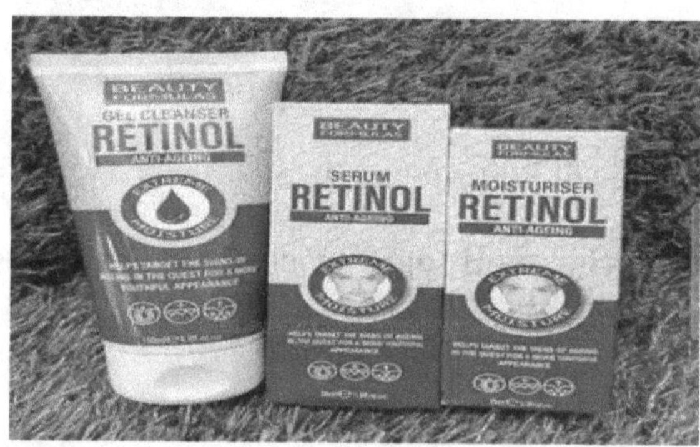

In this chapter, we will explore specialized DIY recipes for anti-aging skincare. These formulas are designed to help reduce the signs of aging and keep your skin looking youthful and vibrant.

1. Hydrating Rosehip Seed Oil Serum

Ingredients:

- 2 tablespoons of rosehip seed oil

- 1 tablespoon of jojoba oil

- 5-10 drops of frankincense essential oil

- 5-10 drops of rose essential oil

Instructions:

1. In a small bottle, combine the rosehip seed oil, jojoba oil, frankincense essential oil, and rose essential oil.

2. Shake well to blend the oils.

3. Apply a few drops of the serum to your face and neck after cleansing, both morning and night.

Benefits: Rosehip seed oil is rich in antioxidants and vitamins, while frankincense and rose essential oils promote skin rejuvenation.

2. DIY Vitamin C Face Mask

Ingredients:

- 1 tablespoon of vitamin C powder

- 1 tablespoon of honey

- 1 tablespoon of plain yogurt

Instructions:

1. Mix the vitamin C powder, honey, and yogurt in a bowl to form a paste.

2. Apply the mask to your face, avoiding the eye area.

3. Leave it on for 15-20 minutes.

4. Rinse with lukewarm water and follow with your regular skincare routine.

Benefits: Vitamin C brightens and boosts collagen production, honey hydrates, and yogurt soothes.

3. Retinol-Infused Night Cream

Ingredients:

- 2 tablespoons of shea butter

- 1 tablespoon of jojoba oil

- 1 teaspoon of vitamin E oil

- 1/2 teaspoon of retinol cream (available at drugstores)

Instructions:

1. In a double boiler, melt the shea butter and jojoba oil.

2. Remove from heat and stir in the vitamin E oil and retinol cream.

3. Allow the mixture to cool and solidify.

4. Apply the night cream to your face and neck before bedtime.

Benefits: Shea butter and jojoba oil moisturize, vitamin E provides antioxidant protection, and retinol helps reduce the appearance of fine lines and wrinkles.

4. Green Tea and Aloe Vera Eye Gel

Ingredients:

- 1/4 cup of brewed green tea (cooled)

- 1/4 cup of aloe vera gel

- 1/2 teaspoon of vitamin E oil

Instructions:

1. Mix the brewed green tea, aloe vera gel, and vitamin E oil in a small container.

2. Apply a small amount of the gel around your eyes, avoiding direct contact with the eyes.

3. Gently pat it into the skin.

4. Use it morning and night as part of your skincare routine.

Benefits: Green tea is rich in antioxidants, aloe vera soothes, and vitamin E nourishes the delicate skin around the eyes.

These specialized anti-aging skincare recipes are like elixirs for your skin, helping you combat the signs of aging and maintain a youthful complexion. As you incorporate these formulas into your skincare routine, remember the importance of self-care and the rejuvenation it brings to your skin and spirit.

B. Acne-Fighting Solutions

In this section, we will explore specialized DIY recipes for acne-fighting skincare. These solutions are designed to help combat acne and promote clear, healthy skin.

1. Tea Tree Oil Acne Spot Treatment

Ingredients:

- 1 tablespoon of jojoba oil

- 5-10 drops of tea tree essential oil

Instructions:

1. In a small bottle, combine the jojoba oil and tea tree essential oil.

2. Mix well.

3. Apply a small amount of the mixture directly to acne spots using a clean cotton swab.

4. Leave it on overnight.

5. Rinse off in the morning and follow your regular skincare routine.

Benefits: Tea tree oil has antibacterial properties that help reduce acne, while jojoba oil moisturizes and soothes the skin.

2. Honey and Cinnamon Face Mask

Ingredients:

- 2 tablespoons of honey

- 1 teaspoon of cinnamon powder

Instructions:

1. Mix the honey and cinnamon powder in a bowl to create a paste.

2. Apply the mask to your face, avoiding the eye area.

3. Leave it on for 15-20 minutes.

4. Rinse with lukewarm water and follow with your regular skincare routine.

Benefits: Honey has antibacterial properties and moisturizes the skin, while cinnamon helps reduce inflammation and acne.

3. DIY Salicylic Acid Toner

Ingredients:

- 1/4 cup of witch hazel

- 1/4 cup of distilled water

- 2 tablespoons of apple cider vinegar

- 2 aspirin tablets (crushed)

Instructions:

1. Mix the witch hazel, distilled water, and apple cider vinegar in a bottle.

2. Add the crushed aspirin tablets to the mixture and shake well until dissolved.

3. Use a cotton pad to apply the toner to your clean face, focusing on acne-prone areas.

4. Follow with your regular skincare routine.

Benefits: Salicylic acid (derived from aspirin) exfoliates and unclogs pores, witch hazel tightens and tones, and apple cider vinegar balances skin's pH.

4. Turmeric and Yogurt Face Mask

Ingredients:

- 1 tablespoon of plain yogurt

- 1/2 teaspoon of turmeric powder

Instructions:

1. Mix the yogurt and turmeric powder in a bowl to form a paste.

2. Apply the mask to your face, avoiding the eye area.

3. Leave it on for 10-15 minutes.

4. Rinse with lukewarm water and follow with your regular skincare routine.

Benefits: Turmeric has anti-inflammatory and antibacterial properties, while yogurt soothes and moisturizes the skin.

These specialized acne-fighting skincare recipes are like allies in your battle for clear, healthy skin. As you incorporate these solutions into your skincare routine, remember the importance of self-care and the empowerment it brings in dealing with acne and maintaining your skin's well-being.

C. Eczema and Psoriasis Relief

In this section, we will explore specialized DIY recipes for providing relief from eczema and psoriasis, two common skin conditions that can cause discomfort and irritation.

1. Soothing Oatmeal Bath

Ingredients:

- 1 cup of colloidal oatmeal

- Warm bathwater

Instructions:

1. Sprinkle the colloidal oatmeal into your warm bathwater.

2. Stir the water to disperse the oatmeal evenly.

3. Soak in the oatmeal bath for 15-20 minutes.

4. Gently pat your skin dry with a soft towel, and avoid rubbing.

Benefits: Colloidal oatmeal is known for its soothing properties, helping to relieve itching and inflammation associated with eczema and psoriasis.

2. Calming Aloe Vera Gel

Ingredients:

- Fresh aloe vera gel (obtained from an aloe leaf)

Instructions:

1. Cut open an aloe leaf and extract the fresh gel from inside.

2. Apply the aloe vera gel directly to affected areas of your skin.

3. Allow it to air dry.

4. Repeat this process several times a day as needed for relief.

Benefits: Aloe vera has anti-inflammatory and moisturizing properties, making it effective in soothing irritated skin.

3. Coconut Oil and Lavender Balm

Ingredients:

- 1/4 cup of coconut oil

- 10-15 drops of lavender essential oil

Instructions:

1. In a small container, mix the coconut oil and lavender essential oil.

2. Allow the mixture to cool and solidify (you can refrigerate it for faster solidification).

3. Apply the balm to affected areas as needed to soothe dry and itchy skin.

Benefits: Coconut oil moisturizes and lavender essential oil provides a calming effect while helping with skin irritation.

4. Chamomile and Jojoba Oil Lotion

Ingredients

- 1/4 cup of chamomile-infused jojoba oil (place dried chamomile flowers in jojoba oil and let sit for a few weeks)

- 1 tablespoon of beeswax pellets

Instructions:

1. In a double boiler, melt the chamomile-infused jojoba oil and beeswax pellets.

2. Remove from heat and allow it to cool and solidify.

3. Apply the chamomile and jojoba oil lotion to affected areas to provide relief from dry and irritated skin.

Benefits: Chamomile is known for its anti-inflammatory and soothing properties, while jojoba oil moisturizes and nourishes the skin.

These specialized skincare recipes are like gentle allies in your journey to find relief from eczema and psoriasis. As you use these solutions to care for your skin, remember the importance of self-compassion and the comfort it brings in managing these conditions and maintaining the well-being of your skin.

D. Natural Remedies for Skin Conditions

In this section, we will explore specialized DIY recipes for addressing various skin conditions using natural remedies. These solutions aim to provide relief and promote skin health for a variety of concerns.

1. Calendula and Lavender Healing Salve

Ingredients:

- 1/4 cup of calendula-infused olive oil (place dried calendula petals in olive oil and let sit for a few weeks)

- 2 tablespoons of beeswax pellets

- 10-15 drops of lavender essential oil

Instructions:

1. In a double boiler, melt the calendula-infused olive oil and beeswax pellets.

2. Remove from heat and add the lavender essential oil.

3. Allow the mixture to cool and solidify.

4. Apply the healing salve to affected areas to soothe skin irritations and minor wounds.

Benefits: Calendula is known for its anti-inflammatory and wound-healing properties, while lavender essential oil provides calming relief.

2. Cooling Cucumber and Aloe Vera Gel

Ingredients:

- 1/2 cucumber (peeled and blended)

- 2 tablespoons of aloe vera gel

Instructions:

1. Blend the peeled cucumber until you have a smooth paste.

2. Mix the cucumber paste with aloe vera gel.

3. Apply the cooling gel to sunburned or irritated skin for relief.

Benefits: Cucumber soothes and hydrates, while aloe vera provides a cooling and moisturizing effect.

3. Turmeric and Manuka Honey Face Mask

Ingredients:

- 1 teaspoon of turmeric powder

- 1 tablespoon of Manuka honey

Instructions:

1. Mix the turmeric powder and Manuka honey in a bowl to create a paste.

2. Apply the mask to your face, avoiding the eye area.

3. Leave it on for 10-15 minutes.

4. Rinse with lukewarm water and follow with your regular skincare routine.

Benefits: Turmeric has anti-inflammatory and antimicrobial properties, while Manuka honey helps soothe and moisturize the skin.

4. Witch Hazel and Lavender Toner for Irritated Skin

Ingredients:

- 1/4 cup of witch hazel

- 1/4 cup of rosewater

- 10-15 drops of lavender essential oil

Instructions:

1. Mix the witch hazel, rosewater, and lavender essential oil in a bottle.

2. Shake well before each use.

3. Apply the toner to irritated skin using a cotton pad.

4. Follow with your regular skincare routine.

Benefits: Witch hazel has anti-inflammatory properties, rosewater soothes, and lavender essential oil provides calming relief.

These natural remedies for various skin conditions are like gifts from nature to help you address specific concerns and maintain the health and comfort of your skin. As you incorporate these solutions into your skincare routine, remember the importance of self-care and the empowerment it brings in caring for your skin.

Chapter IX:

Aromatherapy and Skincare

A. Introduction to Aromatherapy

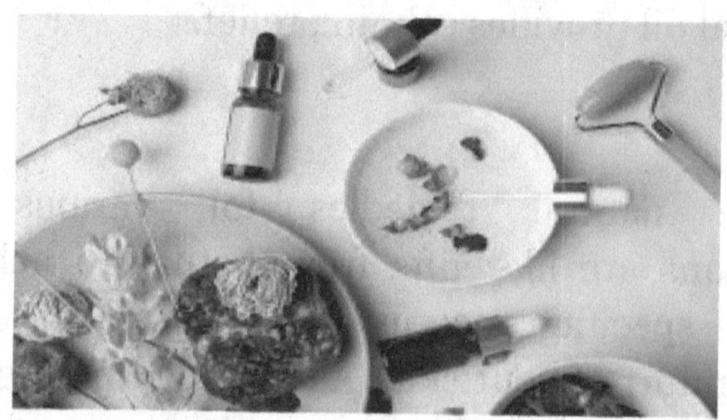

In this chapter, we will explore the fascinating world of aromatherapy and its synergy with skincare. Aromatherapy is the practice of using essential oils and aromatic compounds from plants to enhance physical and emotional well-being. When applied to skincare, aromatherapy can elevate your skincare routine to a holistic and therapeutic experience.

1. The Essence of Aromatherapy

Aromatherapy, often referred to as essential oil therapy, has been used for centuries in various cultures for its therapeutic properties. It harnesses the aromatic essence of plants, flowers, and herbs to promote health and well-being. These natural essences are extracted from various plant parts, including leaves, flowers, bark, and roots, through processes like steam distillation or cold pressing.

2. The Power of Essential Oils

Essential oils are the heart and soul of aromatherapy. They are highly concentrated plant extracts, each with its unique scent and therapeutic benefits. Some essential oils are known for their skin-loving properties, making them valuable additions to skincare products. For example, lavender oil soothes and calms the skin, while tea tree oil has powerful antibacterial properties.

3. The Marriage of Aromatherapy and Skincare

When incorporated into skincare, aromatherapy can transform your routine into a sensory journey that nurtures both your skin and your spirit. The benefits of this marriage include:

- **Enhanced Mood:** Aromatherapy can positively influence your emotions and mental state. Inhaling the aroma of essential oils can uplift your mood, reduce stress, and promote relaxation.

- **Improved Skin Health:** Many essential oils offer specific benefits for the skin. They can help soothe irritation, balance oil production, and promote a healthy complexion.

- **Holistic Wellness:** Aromatherapy aligns with the concept of holistic wellness, addressing not only physical but also emotional and mental aspects of well-being. This holistic approach can lead to a deeper sense of self-care.

4. Safety First

While essential oils have numerous benefits, it's crucial to use them safely, especially in skincare. Essential oils are potent and should be diluted before applying to the skin. Always perform a patch test to check for allergies or sensitivities. Additionally, consult with a qualified aromatherapist or skincare professional if you have specific concerns or conditions.

As we delve deeper into the world of aromatherapy and skincare in this chapter, you will discover how to harness the therapeutic potential of essential oils in your skincare routine. It's a journey that combines nature's wisdom with self-care, allowing you to embrace the healing power of aromatherapy for your skin and soul.

B. Essential Oil Blends for Skincare

In this section, we will explore essential oil blends specifically crafted to enhance your skincare routine. These blends harness the therapeutic properties of essential oils to address various skin concerns and promote healthy, radiant skin.

1. Radiant Skin Blend for All Skin Types

Ingredients:

- 3 drops of lavender essential oil

- 2 drops of frankincense essential oil

- 2 drops of geranium essential oil

- 1 ounce of a carrier oil (e.g., jojoba, almond, or rosehip seed oil)

Instructions:

1. Mix the lavender, frankincense, and geranium essential oils with your chosen carrier oil in a dark glass bottle.

2. Shake well to blend the oils thoroughly.

3. Apply a few drops of the blend to your face and neck after cleansing and before moisturizing.

Benefits: Lavender soothes, frankincense rejuvenates, and geranium balances the skin's oil production, resulting in a radiant complexion.

2. Acne-Fighting Blend

Ingredients:

- 3 drops of tea tree essential oil

- 2 drops of lavender essential oil

- 2 drops of rosemary essential oil

- 1 ounce of a carrier oil (e.g., jojoba or grapeseed oil)

Instructions:

1. Mix the tea tree, lavender, and rosemary essential oils with your chosen carrier oil in a dark glass bottle.

2. Shake well to blend the oils thoroughly.

3. Apply a small amount of the blend to acne-prone areas after cleansing.

Benefits: Tea tree oil fights acne-causing bacteria, lavender soothes, and rosemary reduces inflammation, making this blend effective for acne-prone skin.

3. Anti-Aging Elixir

Ingredients:

- 3 drops of rose essential oil

- 2 drops of frankincense essential oil

- 1 drop of carrot seed essential oil

- 1 ounce of a carrier oil (e.g., rosehip seed or argan oil)

Instructions:

1. Mix the rose, frankincense, and carrot seed essential oils with your chosen carrier oil in a dark glass bottle.

2. Shake well to blend the oils thoroughly.

3. Apply a few drops of the elixir to your face and neck after cleansing and before moisturizing.

Benefits: Rose oil hydrates and tones, frankincense promotes skin rejuvenation, and carrot seed oil supports skin elasticity, all contributing to a youthful complexion.

4. Calming Sensitivity Blend

Ingredients:

- 3 drops of chamomile essential oil

- 2 drops of lavender essential oil

- 2 drops of rose essential oil

- 1 ounce of a carrier oil (e.g., jojoba or avocado oil)

Instructions:

1. Mix the chamomile, lavender, and rose essential oils with your chosen carrier oil in a dark glass bottle.

2. Shake well to blend the oils thoroughly.

3. Apply a few drops of the blend to sensitive or irritated areas for soothing relief.

Benefits: Chamomile calms irritation, lavender soothes, and rose oil provides gentle care for sensitive skin.

These essential oil blends are like personalized skincare elixirs, designed to address specific skin concerns and enhance the health and beauty of your skin. As you incorporate these blends into your skincare routine, remember the importance of self-care and the holistic well-being they bring to your skin and spirit.

C. Creating a Relaxing Skincare Routine

In this section, we will explore how to create a soothing and relaxing skincare routine infused with the power of aromatherapy. A well-crafted routine not only cares for your skin but also nurtures your mind, helping you unwind and destress after a long day.

1. Evening Aromatherapy Cleanse

Begin your relaxing skincare routine in the evening with an aromatherapy cleanse. Use a gentle, natural cleanser suitable for your skin type. Consider adding a few drops of lavender or chamomile essential oil to your cleanser to enhance the calming and soothing effects.

2. Steam Facial

After cleansing, treat yourself to a steam facial. Boil water and pour it into a bowl. Add a few drops of your favorite calming essential oil, such as lavender or rose, to the hot water. Drape a towel over your head and the bowl, creating a steam tent. Close your eyes, inhale deeply, and let the steam envelop your face for 5-10 minutes. This step not only cleanses your pores but also provides relaxation.

3. Exfoliation with Aromatherapy

Choose a gentle exfoliator suitable for your skin type. Mix it with a drop or two of a refreshing essential oil like lemon or eucalyptus. Gently exfoliate your skin in circular motions, paying attention to areas prone to dryness or congestion.

4. Aromatherapy Face Mask

Apply a soothing aromatherapy face mask. Mix a ready-made mask with a few drops of your favorite essential oil or create a DIY mask using natural ingredients like honey, yogurt, or oatmeal. Lavender, chamomile, and rose essential oils work wonders in masks for relaxation.

5. Relaxing Facial Massage

Take a few moments to massage your face with an aromatherapy-infused facial oil. Create a blend using a carrier oil like jojoba or almond oil and add a drop or two of a calming essential oil such as lavender or bergamot. Gently massage your face and neck using upward, circular motions.

6. Aromatherapy Toner

Apply an aromatherapy toner to balance your skin's pH and provide a refreshing sensation. Use a rosewater or chamomile-infused toner with added drops of your chosen essential oil.

7. Nourishing Night Serum

Finish your evening routine with a nourishing night serum. Create a blend using a carrier oil like rosehip seed or argan oil and add a drop or two of a rejuvenating essential oil such as frankincense or myrrh. Apply the serum to your face and neck, gently massaging it in.

8. Bedtime Aromatherapy Ritual

As a final step, engage in an aromatherapy bedtime ritual. Use a diffuser to fill your bedroom with the soothing scent of lavender, chamomile, or cedarwood essential oil. This promotes relaxation and sets the stage for a peaceful night's sleep.

By incorporating aromatherapy into your skincare routine, you transform it into a holistic self-care experience that nourishes both your skin and your soul. These moments of relaxation and pampering can help you unwind, reduce stress, and enhance your overall well-being. Remember that self-care is an essential part of maintaining healthy and radiant skin.

Chapter X:
Customizing Your Skincare

A. Adapting Recipes to Your Skin Type

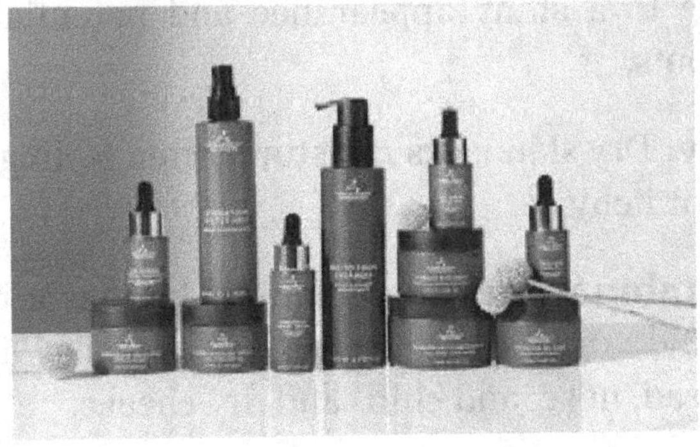

In this chapter, we will explore the art of customizing skincare recipes to cater to your unique skin type and its changing needs. Every person's skin is different, and understanding your skin type is crucial for creating effective and tailored skincare products.

1. Identifying Your Skin Type

Before you can customize your skincare, you need to identify your skin type. Common skin types include:

- **Oily:** Oily skin tends to produce excess sebum, leading to a shiny appearance and potential acne breakouts.

- **Dry:** Dry skin lacks moisture, often feeling tight, flaky, or itchy.

- **Combination:** Combination skin has a mix of oily and dry areas, typically an oily T-zone (forehead, nose, and chin) and dry cheeks.

- **Sensitive:** Sensitive skin is prone to irritation, redness, and discomfort.

- **Normal:** Normal skin is well-balanced, neither too oily nor too dry.

2. Customizing Cleansers

- For Oily Skin: Choose a foaming cleanser with ingredients like salicylic acid to control oil.

- For Dry Skin: Opt for a hydrating, creamy cleanser with ingredients like hyaluronic acid.

- For Sensitive Skin: Use a gentle, fragrance-free cleanser to avoid irritation.

3. Customizing Moisturizers

- For Oily Skin: Select a lightweight, oil-free moisturizer with ingredients like niacinamide.

- For Dry Skin: Choose a rich, hydrating moisturizer with ingredients like shea butter or ceramides.

- For Sensitive Skin: Look for a hypoallergenic, fragrance-free moisturizer with soothing ingredients like aloe vera.

4. Customizing Toners

- For Oily Skin: Use a toner with witch hazel or salicylic acid to control oil.

- For Dry Skin: Opt for a hydrating toner with ingredients like glycerin.

- For Sensitive Skin: Use a soothing, alcohol-free toner with chamomile or rosewater.

5. Customizing Face Masks

- For Oily Skin: Try clay masks with ingredients like kaolin or bentonite to absorb excess oil.

- For Dry Skin: Use hydrating masks with ingredients like honey or hyaluronic acid.

- For Sensitive Skin: Choose gentle, fragrance-free masks with oatmeal or aloe vera.

6. Customizing Serums

- For Oily Skin: Use serums with niacinamide or tea tree oil to control oil and minimize pores.

- For Dry Skin: Look for serums containing hyaluronic acid or ceramides for added hydration.

- For Sensitive Skin: Use serums with soothing ingredients like calendula or chamomile.

7. Customizing Essential Oil Blends

If you enjoy aromatherapy and essential oil blends, adapt them to suit your skin type. For example, add lavender or rose oil for dry skin, tea tree or eucalyptus for oily skin, or chamomile for sensitive skin.

8. Monitoring and Adjusting

Remember that your skin's needs can change with factors like the seasons, age, and lifestyle. Regularly assess your skin's condition and adjust your skincare routine accordingly. Be cautious about introducing new products and always perform patch tests.

Customizing your skincare routine to your specific skin type ensures that you provide the right care and achieve the best results. By understanding your skin's unique characteristics and adapting your products accordingly, you can maintain healthy, balanced, and radiant skin throughout your skincare journey.

B. Scent and Texture Personalization

In this section, we will explore the delightful aspect of personalizing your skincare routine through scent and texture preferences. Tailoring the sensory experience of your skincare products can make your routine more enjoyable and gratifying.

1. Customizing Scents

The scent of your skincare products can significantly influence your overall experience. Here's how you can personalize scents:

- **Fragrance-Free:** If you prefer products without added fragrance, choose unscented or fragrance-free options, especially if you have sensitive skin.

- **Essential Oils:** Incorporate essential oils into your routine to add pleasing natural scents. For example, lavender, rose, or chamomile essential oils offer calming aromas, while citrus oils like orange or lemon provide refreshing notes.

- **Aromatherapy Blends:** Experiment with aromatherapy by blending essential oils that resonate with your mood. Create a relaxing bedtime blend or an invigorating morning blend to elevate your skincare ritual.

2. Personalizing Textures

The texture of your skincare products can enhance the application experience. Customize textures based on your preferences:

- **Lightweight:** Opt for lightweight lotions or gels if you prefer a product that absorbs quickly and doesn't leave a heavy feeling on your skin. These are great for those with oily or combination skin.

- **Creamy and Nourishing:** Choose rich, creamy textures for deep hydration and comfort, ideal for dry or mature skin. These products provide a protective barrier and a luxurious feel.

- **Gel-Based:** Gel-based products are refreshing and can be soothing for sensitive or irritated skin. They're also excellent choices for hot and humid climates.

- Whipped or Mousse: These textures feel airy and fun, adding an element of indulgence to your skincare routine. They're great for those who enjoy a sensory experience.

3. Mixing and Matching

Don't hesitate to mix and match textures and scents within your routine. For example, you can use a lightweight, citrus-scented serum in the morning to invigorate your senses, and a rich, lavender-infused night cream before bed for relaxation.

4. Seasonal Adaptation

Consider adjusting your skincare textures and scents with the changing seasons. Lighter textures may be preferred during the summer months, while richer products can provide comfort during the winter. Opt for scents that align with the season, such as floral notes in spring and earthy or warm scents in fall.

5. Mindful Application

As you apply your customized products, take a moment to indulge in the sensory experience. Inhale the scents, feel the textures, and let the process become a mindful ritual that nurtures not only your skin but also your well-being.

Personalizing the scent and texture of your skincare products allows you to enjoy a sensory journey tailored to your preferences. By infusing your skincare routine with scents and textures that resonate with you, you can elevate your self-care experience and create a daily ritual that brings joy and satisfaction to your skincare journey.

C. Troubleshooting Common Issues

In this section, we will delve into troubleshooting common skincare issues and how to adapt your routine to address them effectively. Skincare isn't always smooth sailing, but with the right adjustments, you can overcome challenges and maintain healthy, radiant skin.

1. Breakouts and Acne

Troubleshooting Tips:

- For breakouts, use products containing salicylic acid or benzoyl peroxide.

- Avoid over-cleansing, which can strip your skin and exacerbate breakouts.

- Ensure that your skincare routine includes a non-comedogenic moisturizer to keep your skin hydrated without clogging pores.

2. Dry and Flaky Skin

Troubleshooting Tips:

- Opt for a gentle, hydrating cleanser.

- Add a hyaluronic acid serum to your routine to boost moisture.

- Choose a rich, emollient moisturizer and consider using a humidifier in dry environments.

3. Sensitivity and Redness

Troubleshooting Tips:

- Use fragrance-free and hypoallergenic products.

- Incorporate soothing ingredients like aloe vera, chamomile, or niacinamide.

- Apply sunscreen daily to protect your skin from UV damage, which can worsen sensitivity.

4. Excessive Oiliness

Troubleshooting Tips:

- Use a gentle cleanser twice daily to remove excess oil and impurities.

- Incorporate a lightweight, oil-free moisturizer to maintain hydration without adding extra oil.

- Consider using blotting papers throughout the day to manage shine.

5.Uneven Skin Tone and Hyperpigmentation

Troubleshooting Tips:

- Integrate a vitamin C serum into your routine to brighten the skin.

- Apply a broad-spectrum sunscreen daily to prevent further hyperpigmentation.

- Consult a dermatologist for professional treatments like chemical peels or laser therapy if needed.

6. Fine Lines and Wrinkles

Troubleshooting Tips:

- Use a retinol or retinoid product to promote collagen production.

- Ensure your routine includes a moisturizer with hydrating ingredients.

- Be consistent with sunscreen to prevent further sun damage.

7. Clogged Pores and Blackheads

Troubleshooting Tips:

- Consider incorporating an exfoliating product with salicylic acid or glycolic acid.

- Use a clay mask once a week to help draw out impurities.

- Avoid excessive scrubbing, as it can worsen the issue.

8. Allergic Reactions or Irritation

Troubleshooting Tips:

- Identify and eliminate the product causing the reaction.

- Switch to a minimalistic routine with gentle, fragrance-free products.

- Consult a dermatologist if the reaction persists or worsens.

9. Seasonal Adjustments

Remember that your skin's needs may change with the seasons. Adapt your routine accordingly, opting for lighter products in hot weather and richer products during colder months.

10. Professional Guidance

If you encounter persistent or severe skincare issues, consider consulting a dermatologist. They can provide tailored advice and treatments to address specific concerns.

Troubleshooting common skincare issues is a valuable skill that allows you to adapt and refine your routine as needed. By addressing challenges head-on and making informed adjustments, you can achieve and maintain healthy, beautiful skin.

Chapter XI:

Sustainability and Ethical Practices

A. Choosing Sustainable Ingredients

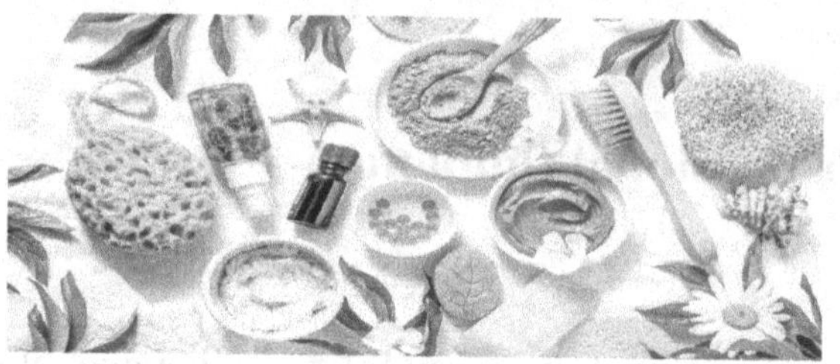

In this chapter, we will explore the importance of choosing sustainable ingredients for your skincare products and how it contributes to ethical and eco-conscious practices in the beauty industry.

1. The Significance of Sustainability

Sustainability in skincare involves selecting ingredients and sourcing practices that minimize negative environmental impacts. It also promotes ethical treatment of workers and supports fair trade.

2. Ethical Ingredient Sourcing

- **Fair Trade:** Choose ingredients sourced from fair trade cooperatives or organizations. This ensures fair wages and working conditions for the people involved in ingredient production.

- **Cruelty-Free:** Opt for ingredients and products that are cruelty-free, meaning they were not tested on animals. Look for certifications from organizations like Leaping Bunny or PETA.

3. Sustainable Ingredient Choices

- **Organic Ingredients:** Select organic ingredients when possible. Organic farming practices reduce chemical pesticide use and promote soil health.

- **Local Sourcing:** Choose locally sourced ingredients to support your community and reduce the carbon footprint associated with transportation.

- **Wildcrafted Ingredients:** Some ingredients are sustainably harvested from the wild, respecting natural ecosystems. Ensure that wildcrafting is done responsibly and without harm to the environment.

- **Certifications:** Look for certifications such as USDA Organic or Ecocert, which indicate sustainable and organic ingredient sourcing.

4. Ingredient Transparency

- Read Labels: Familiarize yourself with ingredient labels to identify harmful chemicals or unsustainable components. Avoid ingredients like microplastics or palm oil, which can contribute to environmental issues.

- Research Suppliers: Investigate the ethical practices of ingredient suppliers and manufacturers. Companies that prioritize sustainability often provide transparency about their sourcing.

5. DIY Skincare and Sustainability

If you create your skincare products, you have control over the ingredients you use. Consider sourcing eco-friendly packaging, using minimal preservatives, and supporting sustainable ingredient suppliers.

6. Reducing Waste

- Minimalist Formulas: Design skincare recipes with fewer ingredients to reduce waste and the risk of allergens.

- Eco-Friendly Packaging: Choose recyclable or biodegradable packaging for your skincare products. Encourage customers to recycle or reuse containers.

7. Supporting Sustainable Brands

Consider purchasing skincare products from brands with strong sustainability and ethical practices. Your consumer choices can influence the industry and encourage responsible practices.

8. Educate and Advocate

Spread awareness about sustainable skincare practices within your community and online. Advocate for ethical sourcing, eco-conscious packaging, and the use of sustainable ingredients.

Choosing sustainable ingredients for your skincare products is a powerful step toward supporting ethical and eco-conscious practices in the beauty industry. By prioritizing sustainability, you contribute to a healthier planet and promote positive changes in the skincare industry as a whole.

B. Reducing Packaging Waste

In this section, we will explore strategies to reduce packaging waste in your skincare products, contributing to more eco-conscious and sustainable practices.

1. Minimalist Packaging

- **Simplified Designs:** Embrace minimalist packaging designs that use fewer materials. Streamline the shape and structure of your containers.

- **Less Printing:** Reduce the amount of printing on packaging to minimize ink usage and make recycling easier.

2. Eco-Friendly Materials

- **Recycled Materials:** Choose packaging made from recycled materials whenever possible. Look for containers made from recycled glass or plastic.

-**Biodegradable Options:** Explore biodegradable packaging materials like compostable paper or plant-based plastics.

- **Refillable Containers:** Offer refillable packaging options, allowing customers to reuse their containers. This reduces the need for new packaging with each purchase.

3. Sustainable Labels

- Labels with Eco Inks: Use labels with eco-friendly inks that are less harmful to the environment.

- Label Placement: Position labels on packaging to facilitate easy removal, which can improve recycling efforts.

4. Packaging Reduction

- Concentrated Products: Develop concentrated formulas that require smaller packaging due to higher potency.

- Multi-Use Products: Create products with multiple uses, reducing the number of separate items customers need.

5. Reusable Packaging

- Packaging as a Keepsake: Design packaging that customers may want to keep and reuse. For example, a beautifully crafted glass jar could be repurposed for other purposes.

- Education: Encourage customers to find creative ways to reuse or upcycle your product packaging, reducing its environmental impact.

6. Package-Free Options

- Naked Products: Consider offering "naked" or package-free options, where the product itself serves as its own packaging.

7. Collaborate with Recycling Programs

- Educate Customers: Provide information to customers about how to properly recycle your product packaging.

- Collaborate with Recycling Initiatives:
Partner with local recycling programs or
organizations to ensure that your packaging is
disposed of responsibly.

8. Responsible Shipping

- Eco-Friendly Shipping Materials: Use
sustainable shipping materials, such as recycled
cardboard boxes and biodegradable packing
peanuts.

- Minimal Packaging: Avoid over-packaging
when shipping products. Use only the necessary
materials to protect the items during transit.

9. Consumer Education

- Inform Customers: Educate your customers
about the importance of recycling and proper
disposal of skincare product packaging.

- **Incentives:** Consider offering incentives to customers who return empty product containers for recycling.

By adopting these strategies to reduce packaging waste, you can make a significant contribution to sustainability in the skincare industry. These practices not only benefit the environment but also align with the growing consumer demand for eco-conscious and responsible packaging solutions.

C. Supporting Ethical Brands

In this section, we will discuss the significance of supporting ethical brands in the skincare industry and how your choices as a consumer or skincare creator can promote ethical practices.

1. Understanding Ethical Skincare Brands

- Values Alignment: Seek brands whose values align with your own, such as those committed to sustainability, cruelty-free practices, fair wages, and ethical sourcing.

- Transparency: Look for brands that are transparent about their ingredient sourcing, production processes, and ethical initiatives.

2. Research and Due Diligence

- Investigate Brands: Before purchasing skincare products, research the brands behind them. Read about their ethical practices, certifications, and sustainability efforts.

- Independent Reviews: Explore reviews and testimonials from other consumers to gain insights into a brand's reputation and commitment to ethics.

3. Cruelty-Free Products

- Choose Cruelty-Free: Support brands that do not conduct animal testing and have cruelty-free certifications. These brands prioritize the welfare of animals in product development.

4. Sustainable Sourcing

- Sustainable Ingredients: Prefer brands that source ingredients sustainably and have certifications like USDA Organic or Fair Trade to ensure ethical practices.

- Eco-Conscious Packaging: Look for brands that use eco-friendly and recyclable packaging materials to minimize environmental impact.

5. Ethical Labor Practices

- **Fair Wages:** Support brands that pay fair wages to workers involved in the production process, from ingredient sourcing to manufacturing.

- **Ethical Supply Chains:** Choose brands that maintain ethical supply chains, ensuring that workers' rights and well-being are protected.

6. Community Engagement

- **Social Responsibility:** Seek brands that engage with and contribute positively to the communities where they operate. This may include initiatives like supporting local charities or environmental conservation efforts.

7. Advocate for Ethical Practices

- **Spread Awareness:** Share information about ethical skincare brands and the importance of supporting them with your friends and family.

- **Consumer Influence:** Recognize the influence consumers have in shaping the industry. Your purchasing choices send a clear message to brands about your priorities.

8. Collaborate with Ethical Brands

- **Partnerships:** If you create skincare products, consider collaborating with ethical ingredient suppliers and eco-conscious packaging companies to align your brand with ethical practices.

9. Stay Informed

- **Industry Updates:** Stay informed about the latest developments in ethical skincare practices and industry standards. This knowledge can guide your choices.

By consciously choosing to support ethical skincare brands, you contribute to the growth of a more responsible and sustainable beauty industry. Your consumer choices can help drive positive change, encourage ethical practices, and promote a brighter future for skincare that values both people and the planet.

Chapter XII:

Safety and Allergies

A. Patch Testing and Safety Precautions

In this chapter, we will explore the critical importance of patch testing and safety precautions when it comes to skincare products. Ensuring the safety and compatibility of skincare products with your skin is paramount to a healthy skincare routine.

1. The Significance of Patch Testing

- **Allergic Reactions:** Patch testing is a method to identify potential allergic reactions or skin sensitivities to new skincare products. It helps prevent adverse skin reactions.

- **Diverse Skin Reactions:** Keep in mind that everyone's skin is unique. What works well for one person may not be suitable for another.

2. How to Perform a Patch Test

- **Select a Small Area:** Choose a small, inconspicuous area on your skin, such as the inside of your wrist or behind your ear.

- Apply the Product: Apply a small amount of the new skincare product to the chosen area. Follow the product's instructions for usage.

- Wait and Observe: Leave the product on the skin for at least 24 hours. During this time, closely monitor the area for any signs of redness, itching, burning, or other adverse reactions.

3. Interpretation of Results

- No Reaction: If there is no adverse reaction after 24 hours, it's generally safe to use the product on your face or body.

- Mild Reaction: If you experience slight redness or mild irritation that resolves quickly, you may choose to proceed with caution. Consider using the product less frequently or in a lower concentration.

- Severe Reaction: If you experience a severe reaction such as intense itching, burning, or hives, discontinue use immediately and wash the area thoroughly. Seek medical attention if necessary.

4. Safety Precautions

- Read Labels: Always read the ingredient list on skincare products. Be aware of any known allergens or ingredients that you have reacted to in the past.

- Introduce One Product at a Time: When incorporating new products into your skincare routine, introduce them one at a time. This makes it easier to identify the source of any adverse reactions.

- Avoid Overuse: Use products as directed, and avoid overusing them, which can lead to skin sensitivity.

- Consult a Dermatologist: If you have a history of skin allergies or sensitivities, or if you experience persistent skin issues, consult a dermatologist for professional guidance.

5. Allergen Awareness

- Common Allergens: Be aware of common skincare allergens, such as fragrances, preservatives *(e.g., parabens)*, and certain essential oils *(e.g., tea tree oil or peppermint oil)*.

- Hypoallergenic Options: Consider hypoallergenic skincare products designed for sensitive skin, as they are formulated to minimize the risk of allergic reactions.

6. Sensitivity to Sun Exposure

- Some skincare ingredients, like alpha hydroxy acids (AHAs) and retinoids, can increase sensitivity to the sun. When using such products, apply sunscreen daily to protect your skin from UV damage.

Patch testing is a simple yet crucial step in maintaining healthy and irritation-free skin. By being diligent about patch testing and following safety precautions, you can make informed decisions about the skincare products you use, reduce the risk of adverse reactions, and enjoy a skincare routine that supports the well-being of your skin.

B. Common Allergens to Watch For

In this section, we will discuss common allergens found in skincare products that you should be aware of to help prevent allergic reactions and skin sensitivities.

1. Fragrances

- Perfumes and Fragrance Oils: Many skincare products contain added fragrances to make them more appealing. However, these fragrances can be a common source of skin irritation and allergic reactions. Look for products labeled *"fragrance-free" or "unscented."*

2. Preservatives

- Parabens: Parabens are a group of synthetic preservatives commonly used in cosmetics and skincare products. Some people may develop allergic reactions or skin sensitivities to parabens. Opt for products labeled *"paraben-free."*

3. Essential Oils

- Tea Tree Oil: While tea tree oil has many potential benefits, it can be a skin irritant for some individuals, especially when used undiluted or in high concentrations.

- Peppermint Oil: Peppermint oil is known for its cooling sensation, but it can be too harsh for sensitive skin and may cause irritation.

- Citrus Oils: Citrus essential oils like lemon or lime can make the skin more sensitive to sunlight, potentially leading to sunburn.

4. Allergenic Ingredients

- Nickel: Some skincare products may contain traces of nickel, which can cause allergic reactions, especially in individuals with nickel allergies.

- Propylene Glycol: This common skincare ingredient can cause skin irritation or contact dermatitis in sensitive individuals.

- Fragrance Allergens: Within the category of fragrances, there are specific allergens known to cause skin reactions, such as limonene, linalool, and citronellol. Check ingredient labels for these substances.

5. Harsh Exfoliants

- **Physical Exfoliants:** Scrubs with coarse particles like apricot kernels can be too abrasive for some skin types and lead to microtears and irritation.

- **Alpha Hydroxy Acids (AHAs):** AHAs like glycolic acid and lactic acid can be beneficial for exfoliation but may cause sensitivity or redness in some individuals. Start with lower concentrations if you're new to AHAs.

6. Sunscreen Ingredients

- **Chemical Sunscreen Ingredients:** Some individuals may experience skin reactions to specific chemical sunscreen ingredients like oxybenzone or avobenzone. Consider trying physical sunscreens (zinc oxide or titanium dioxide) if you have sensitivities.

7. Plant Extracts

- **Aloe Vera:** While aloe vera is known for its soothing properties, some people may be allergic to it. Perform a patch test if you're unsure.

- **Chamomile:** Chamomile is used for its calming effects, but individuals with ragweed allergies may also react to chamomile.

8. Lanolin

- **Lanolin:** Derived from sheep's wool, lanolin is found in some skincare products. It can be a source of skin irritation and allergic reactions in sensitive individuals.

9. Nuts and Nut Oils

- Almond Oil: While almond oil is used in many skincare products, it can be problematic for individuals with nut allergies. Be cautious if you have such allergies.

- Coconut Oil: Though not a nut in the botanical sense, coconut is classified as a tree nut by the FDA. Some people with nut allergies may react to coconut-derived ingredients.

Being aware of these common allergens in skincare products can help you make informed choices and avoid potential allergic reactions or skin sensitivities. Always read ingredient labels carefully and perform patch tests when introducing new products into your skincare routine, especially if you have a history of skin allergies or sensitivities.

C. First Aid for Skincare Mishaps

In this section, we will cover essential first-aid steps to take in case of skincare mishaps or adverse reactions to skincare products. Quick and appropriate actions can help alleviate discomfort and minimize potential damage.

1. Allergic Reaction or Irritation

- **Wash the Affected Area:** If you experience redness, itching, burning, or irritation after applying a skincare product, immediately wash the affected area with lukewarm water and a gentle, fragrance-free cleanser. Pat the skin dry with a clean, soft towel.

- **Discontinue Use:** Stop using the product that caused the reaction. Avoid applying any other products to the irritated area until the skin has calmed down.

- **Apply a Cold Compress:** To reduce swelling and soothe discomfort, you can apply a cold compress or a clean cloth soaked in cold water to the affected area.

- **Topical Hydrocortisone Cream:** If the irritation persists or worsens, consider applying an over-the-counter hydrocortisone cream as directed to reduce inflammation.

- **Seek Medical Advice:** If the reaction is severe, includes blistering, or if you experience difficulty breathing, swelling of the face, lips, or tongue, seek immediate medical attention, as this may indicate an allergic reaction requiring medical intervention.

2. Sunburn

- **Cool Compress:** Apply a cool, damp cloth to the sunburned area to help reduce heat and discomfort.

- **Hydrate:** Drink plenty of water to stay hydrated, as sunburn can dehydrate the body.

- Avoid Further Sun Exposure: Protect the sunburned area from further sun exposure. If you must go outside, wear protective clothing and sunscreen.

- Over-the-Counter Pain Relief: Over-the-counter pain relievers like ibuprofen or aspirin may help reduce pain and inflammation. Follow the package instructions for dosing.

- Aloe Vera: Apply aloe vera gel to the sunburned skin to soothe and moisturize it.

- Avoid Harsh Skincare Products: Avoid using harsh skincare products on sunburned skin. Stick to gentle, fragrance-free moisturizers.

3. Over-Exfoliation or Sensitivity

- Cease Exfoliation: If you've over-exfoliated or your skin feels sensitive, immediately stop using exfoliating products like scrubs or chemical exfoliants.

- Gentle Cleansing: Wash your face with a mild, non-abrasive cleanser and lukewarm water. Avoid hot water and harsh scrubbing.

- Hydration: Apply a gentle, hydrating moisturizer to soothe and restore the skin's moisture barrier.

- Avoid Sun Exposure: Over-exfoliated skin is more sensitive to UV damage, so minimize sun exposure and apply sunscreen if you need to go outside.

- Give Your Skin Time: Let your skin recover by avoiding any irritating products for a few days or longer until it feels normal again.

- Consult a Dermatologist: If you experience persistent irritation or worsening symptoms, consult a dermatologist for professional guidance.

4. Eye Contact with Product

- Rinse Thoroughly: If a skincare product comes into contact with your eyes, rinse them immediately with plenty of lukewarm water for at least 15 minutes.

- Remove Contact Lenses: If you wear contact lenses, remove them before rinsing your eyes.

- Seek Medical Attention: If irritation persists, if the product contains known eye irritants, or if you experience severe discomfort, consult an eye doctor or seek immediate medical attention.

Remember that prevention is the best approach to skincare mishaps. Always perform patch tests when trying new products, read ingredient labels, and be cautious with products containing known allergens. If an adverse reaction occurs, follow the appropriate first-aid steps and seek professional help if necessary.

Chapter XIII:

Conclusion

A. Embracing Natural Beauty

In this final chapter, we reflect on the journey we've taken through *"100 Organic Skincare Recipes: A Comprehensive Guide to Natural Beauty"* and the importance of embracing natural beauty.

1. The Beauty of Natural Ingredients

Throughout this book, we've explored the incredible potential of natural ingredients. From essential oils to herbs and botanicals, these gifts from nature offer not only skincare benefits but also a deeper connection to the world around us. Embracing natural beauty means recognizing the power and simplicity of what the Earth provides.

2. Honoring Individuality

Natural beauty embraces the uniqueness of every individual. No two people have the exact same skin, needs, or preferences. This book has encouraged you to tailor your skincare routine to fit your specific requirements, whether it's addressing concerns like acne, dryness, or sensitivity or simply indulging in self-care rituals that make you feel radiant.

3. Sustainable Practices

Throughout our exploration, we've emphasized the importance of sustainability and ethical practices in skincare. By choosing products and ingredients that align with these values, you not only care for your skin but also contribute to a healthier planet and support ethical standards in the industry.

4. Empowerment Through Knowledge

Knowledge is a powerful tool in the pursuit of natural beauty. Understanding the benefits of organic skincare, recognizing common allergens, and knowing how to troubleshoot skincare issues empowers you to make informed choices that benefit both your skin and overall well-being.

5. Self-Care as a Priority

Embracing natural beauty is more than just skincare; it's a holistic approach to self-care. It's about recognizing that taking time for yourself, indulging in soothing rituals, and nourishing your body and spirit are essential aspects of feeling beautiful inside and out.

6. Celebrating the Journey

As you embark on your natural beauty journey, remember that it's a process. Skincare is not a destination but a lifelong practice of self-love and self-care. Celebrate the small victories and enjoy the journey of discovering what works best for you.

7. Community and Sharing

The beauty of natural skincare is best appreciated when shared. Share your knowledge, experiences, and newfound recipes with friends and family. Encourage others to embrace natural beauty and make conscious choices that benefit themselves and the world around them.

B. Your Journey to Radiant Skin

Your journey to radiant skin has been an exploration of self-care, empowerment, and embracing the beauty of nature. As you conclude this book, take a moment to reflect on the path you've traveled and the steps you've taken toward achieving healthier and more radiant skin.

1. Self-Discovery and Empowerment

- Throughout this journey, you've discovered the unique needs of your skin and learned how to address them with organic and natural ingredients. This newfound knowledge empowers you to make informed choices for your skincare routine.

2. Sustainable and Ethical Beauty

- You've embraced the importance of sustainability and ethical practices in the beauty industry. By choosing eco-conscious products and supporting ethical brands, you've contributed to a brighter and more responsible future for skincare.

3. The Joy of Self-Care

- Self-care has become a central part of your daily life. You've recognized that self-love and self-care are not indulgent luxuries but essential components of overall well-being.

4. Community and Sharing

- Sharing your skincare journey with others has been a source of inspiration and connection. By spreading knowledge and encouraging loved ones to embrace natural beauty, you've become an advocate for healthier choices.

5. The Beauty of Nature

- Above all, you've celebrated the beauty of nature's gifts. From botanical ingredients to essential oils and herbs, you've harnessed the power of the Earth to nourish and rejuvenate your skin.

As you move forward, remember that your journey to radiant skin is ongoing. It's a journey that celebrates your natural beauty, your individuality, and your commitment to self-care and sustainability. Embrace each day as an opportunity to care for yourself, your skin, and the planet. Your radiant skin is a reflection of the care and love you invest in yourself, a testament to the beauty that comes from within.

C. Resources for Further Learning

As you conclude your journey through *"100 Organic Skincare Recipes: A Comprehensive Guide to Natural Beauty,"* here are some valuable resources to continue expanding your knowledge and passion for natural skincare and beauty:

1. Books

- The Green Beauty Guide by Julie Gabriel: A comprehensive guide to green beauty products and DIY recipes.

- Plant-Powered Beauty by Amy Galper and Christina Daigneault: Explore plant-based skincare ingredients and DIY recipes.

- Skin Cleanse by Adina Grigore: An insightful book that delves into the world of natural skincare.

2. Online Communities and Forums

- Connect with like-minded individuals in online communities and forums dedicated to natural skincare and beauty. Websites like Reddit's r/SkincareAddiction or r/DIYBeauty are great places to start.

3. YouTube Channels and Blogs

- Follow beauty influencers and bloggers who specialize in natural skincare and DIY beauty recipes. They often share tutorials, product reviews, and personal experiences.

4. Natural Skincare Courses

- Consider enrolling in online courses or workshops that focus on natural skincare formulation. Many experts offer courses on topics like herbal skincare, essential oil blending, and sustainable beauty practices.

5. Environmental and Ethical Organizations

- Stay informed about sustainability and ethical practices in the beauty industry by following organizations like the Environmental Working Group (EWG) and the Campaign for Safe Cosmetics.

6. Professional Guidance

- If you have specific skin concerns or conditions, consulting a dermatologist or skincare specialist is invaluable. They can provide personalized advice and treatment plans tailored to your needs.

7. Local Herbalists and Apothecaries

- Explore your local community for herbalists or apothecaries who specialize in natural skincare. They often offer workshops and resources for creating herbal remedies.

8. Ingredient Suppliers

- Connect with suppliers of organic and natural skincare ingredients. Many of them provide resources, ingredient descriptions, and educational materials on their websites.

9. Sustainability Organizations

- Stay informed about sustainable practices in skincare by following organizations such as the Sustainable Cosmetics Initiative (SCI).

10. Social Media and Podcasts

- Follow social media accounts and podcasts dedicated to natural skincare, green beauty, and sustainability for regular updates and insights.

Remember that the world of natural skincare is constantly evolving. Continuing to learn and stay informed will help you make informed choices, experiment with new recipes, and deepen your appreciation for the beauty of nature and self-care. Your journey to radiant, natural beauty is a lifelong exploration, and these resources are here to support and inspire you every step of the way.

In closing, *"100 Organic Skincare Recipes: A Comprehensive Guide to Natural Beauty"* has been a journey of exploration and empowerment. Embrace the beauty of natural ingredients, honor your individuality, prioritize sustainability, and remember that self-care is an essential act of self-love. By doing so, you'll not only nurture your skin but also radiate the beauty that comes from within, embracing your natural, authentic self.

Chapter XIV:

Appendices

A. Ingredient Glossary

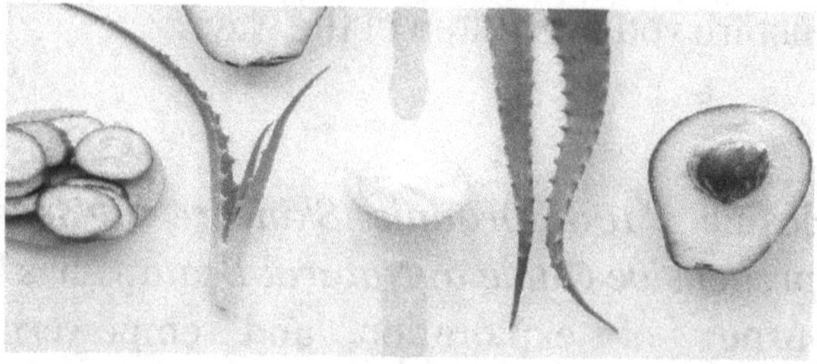

I n this appendix, you will find a comprehensive glossary of common ingredients used in organic skincare recipes. Understanding these ingredients and their benefits will assist you in creating personalized skincare products.

1. Aloe Vera Gel:

- Extracted from the leaves of the aloe vera plant, it soothes and hydrates the skin. Known for its anti-inflammatory and healing properties.

2. Almond Oil:

- A gentle and nourishing oil derived from almonds. It's rich in vitamins and minerals and is often used for its moisturizing properties.

3. Chamomile Extract:

- Known for its calming and anti-inflammatory properties, chamomile extract soothes sensitive skin and can reduce redness.

4. Coconut Oil:

- A versatile oil that moisturizes and conditions the skin. It's often used in various skincare products.

5. Jojoba Oil:

- A lightweight and non-greasy oil that closely resembles the skin's natural sebum. It's known for its moisturizing and balancing effects.

6. Lavender Essential Oil:

- Lavender oil is valued for its calming and soothing properties. It's often used in skincare for its pleasant aroma and potential relaxation benefits.

7. Rosehip Seed Oil:

- Extracted from the seeds of wild rose bushes, this oil is rich in antioxidants and vitamins. It can help with skin rejuvenation and reducing the appearance of scars and fine lines.

8. Shea Butter:

- A creamy, rich butter derived from shea tree nuts. It's highly moisturizing and is often used to soothe dry and sensitive skin.

9. Tea Tree Oil:

- An essential oil known for its antimicrobial and antibacterial properties. It's commonly used for addressing acne and skin blemishes.

10. Witch Hazel:

- Witch hazel is a natural astringent with soothing properties. It's often used to tighten and tone the skin and reduce inflammation.

11. Green Tea Extract:

- Rich in antioxidants, green tea extract can help protect the skin from free radicals and has anti-aging properties.

12. Calendula Oil:

- Derived from marigold flowers, calendula oil is known for its anti-inflammatory and healing properties. It's used to soothe irritated skin.

13. Rosewater:

- A fragrant water made from rose petals. It's known for its hydrating and soothing properties and is often used as a natural toner.

14. Shea Butter:

- Shea butter is a rich and creamy natural fat extracted from shea tree nuts. It's highly moisturizing and is often used in body butters and creams.

15. Vitamin E Oil:

- A powerful antioxidant, vitamin E oil can help protect the skin from environmental damage and support skin health.

16. Argan Oil:

- Derived from argan tree nuts, argan oil is rich in vitamins and fatty acids. It's known for its moisturizing and nourishing properties.

17. Bentonite Clay:

- A natural clay that absorbs excess oil and impurities from the skin. It's often used in facial masks and cleansers.

18. Beeswax:

- A natural wax produced by bees, beeswax is used in skincare products as a thickening agent and emollient.

19. Glycerin:

- A hydrating ingredient that helps to retain moisture in the skin, leaving it soft and supple.

20. Frankincense Essential Oil:

- Known for its soothing and rejuvenating properties, frankincense essential oil is often used in anti-aging skincare formulations.

This glossary serves as a reference for understanding the ingredients used in organic skincare recipes. Each ingredient has its unique benefits, and combining them thoughtfully allows you to create skincare products tailored to your specific needs and preferences.

B. Conversion Charts

In this appendix, you'll find conversion charts to help you accurately measure ingredients when creating your organic skincare recipes. These charts cover various units of measurement commonly used in skincare formulation.

1. Volume Conversions:

- 1 teaspoon (tsp) = 5 milliliters (ml)

- 1 tablespoon (tbsp) = 15 milliliters (ml)

- 1 fluid ounce (oz) = 30 milliliters (ml)

- 1 cup = 240 milliliters (ml)

- 1 pint (pt) = 480 milliliters (ml)

- 1 quart (qt) = 960 milliliters (ml)

- 1 liter (L) = 1,000 milliliters (ml)

2. Weight Conversions:

- 1 gram (g) = 1,000 milligrams (mg)

- 1 ounce (oz) = 28.35 grams (g)

- 1 pound (lb) = 16 ounces (oz) = 453.59 grams (g)

3. Drops and Milliliters Conversion:

- Approximately 20 drops (gtt) = 1 milliliter (ml)

4. Common Ingredient Specific Conversions:

- 1 cup of water = 240 milliliters = 240 grams

- 1 cup of shea butter = 240 milliliters = 240 grams

- 1 cup of coconut oil = 240 milliliters = 240 grams

5. Fahrenheit to Celsius Conversion:

- To convert Fahrenheit (°F) to Celsius (°C), subtract 32 from the Fahrenheit temperature, then multiply the result by 5/9.

- Example: (°F - 32) × 5/9 = °C

6. Celsius to Fahrenheit Conversion:

- To convert Celsius (°C) to Fahrenheit (°F), multiply the Celsius temperature by 9/5 and then add 32.

- Example: (°C × 9/5) + 32 = °F

These conversion charts are essential tools for accurately measuring and using ingredients in your skincare formulations. They ensure that you achieve the desired consistency and effectiveness in your homemade products.

C. Recipe Index

In this section, you'll find an index of all the organic skincare recipes featured in *"100 Organic Skincare Recipes: A Comprehensive Guide to Natural Beauty."* Use this index to quickly locate and reference specific recipes for your skincare needs.

Face Care Recipes:

1. Cleansing Oil for Makeup Removal (Chapter IV, A)

2. Gentle Foaming Cleanser (Chapter IV, A)

3. Honey and Oatmeal Exfoliating Scrub (Chapter IV, A)

4. Soothing Cucumber Toner (Chapter IV, B)

5. Rosewater and Witch Hazel Toner (Chapter IV, B)

6. Vitamin C Serum (Chapter IV, C)

7. Hyaluronic Acid Serum (Chapter IV, C)

8. Avocado and Honey Moisturizer (Chapter IV, C)

9. Detoxifying Clay Mask (Chapter IV, D)

10. Nourishing Yogurt Mask (Chapter IV, D)

Body Care Recipes:

11. Invigorating Citrus Body Wash (Chapter V, A)

12. Sugar and Coconut Oil Scrub (Chapter V, A)

13. Natural Deodorant Paste (Chapter V, B)

14. Luxurious Body Lotion (Chapter V, C)

15. Sunscreen Lotion (Chapter V, D)

16. After-Sun Soothing Gel (Chapter V, D)

Hair Care Recipes:

17. Nourishing Shampoo (Chapter VI, A)

18. Deep Conditioning Hair Mask (Chapter VI, C)

19. Herbal Hair Rinse (Chapter VI, D)

Hand and Foot Care Recipes:

20. Moisturizing Hand Cream (Chapter VII, A)

21. DIY Cuticle Oil (Chapter VII, B)

22. Relaxing Foot Soak (Chapter VII, C)

Specialized Skincare Recipes:

23. Anti-Aging Face Cream (Chapter VIII, A)

24. Acne-Fighting Spot Treatment (Chapter VIII, B)

25. Eczema Relief Balm (Chapter VIII, C)

Aromatherapy and Skincare Recipes:

Customizing Your Skincare Recipes:

Each recipe is designed to address specific skincare concerns and provide you with natural, effective solutions. Use this index to revisit your favorite recipes or discover new ones to incorporate into your skincare routine. Enjoy creating and using these organic skincare products for a radiant and healthy complexion.

Chapter XV:

References and Recommended Reading

In this section, you'll find a list of references and recommended reading materials that have been used as sources of information and inspiration throughout *"100 Organic Skincare Recipes: A Comprehensive Guide to Natural Beauty."* These resources can further deepen your understanding of organic skincare, natural ingredients, and sustainable beauty practices.

1. Books:

- Gabriel, Julie. *The Green Beauty Guide.*

- Galper, Amy, and Christina Daigneault. *Plant-Powered Beauty.*

- Grigore, Adina. *Skin Cleanse.*

- Hammer, Kate. *101 Easy Homemade Products for Your Skin, Health & Home.*

- Rose, Jamie. *Natural Beauty Recipe Book.*

- Stewart, Martha. *Martha Stewart's Beauty Handbook.*

- Worwood, Valerie Ann. *The Complete Book of Essential Oils and Aromatherapy.*

2. Websites and Online Resources:

- Environmental Working Group (EWG): Visit the EWG website for information on skincare product safety and ingredient ratings.

- Campaign for Safe Cosmetics: Explore resources and campaigns advocating for safe cosmetics and skincare products.

- DIY Beauty: Online communities and forums dedicated to DIY beauty and skincare recipes.

3. Scientific Journals:

- Access scientific journals and articles related to skincare, dermatology, and natural ingredients through academic and medical databases.

4. Sustainability Organizations:

- Sustainable Cosmetics Initiative (SCI): Learn more about sustainability initiatives in the cosmetics and skincare industry.

5. Social Media and Blogs:

- Follow beauty influencers, bloggers, and experts in the field of natural skincare on social media platforms and through their blogs for regular updates and insights.

6. Podcasts:

- Explore podcasts dedicated to green beauty, sustainability, and natural skincare for in-depth discussions and interviews with experts.

These references and recommended reading materials are valuable resources for those interested in delving deeper into the world of organic skincare, sustainable beauty practices, and the science behind natural ingredients. They offer a wealth of knowledge to enhance your journey towards healthier and more radiant skin.